Copyright © 2017 Alyson Chugerman
All rights reserved. No part of this book may be reproduced or transmitted in any form or by any means, electronic or mechanical, including photocopying, recording, or by an information storage and retrieval system—except by a reviewer who may quote brief passages in a magazine, newspaper, or online review—without permission in writing from the publisher.

ISBN: 978-0-9972284-4-1

Published by Words In The Works

Eat Real, Live Mindfully, Laugh Often

ATTAIN TRUE HEALTH BODY AND MIND REFRESH

by
ALYSON CHUGERMAN

The Attain True Health
Body and Mind Refresh is
designed to bring awareness
to your physical, emotional
and lifestyle choices and
allow you to gain a deeper
understanding of what
truly works for YOU.

Dedication

To my daughters Haylee and Aubrey who are my inspiration, my motivation and what keeps me going every single day. Their journeys are what set me on my path of helping educate others about the profound impact that sound nutrition and a healthy lifestyle have on our overall health.

DISCLAIMER

Information presented in this publication is not intended to diagnose, treat or cure any particular illness and is not to be used as medical advice. It is meant to raise awareness and understanding of how food and lifestyle can help us reach our own individual health goals.

CONTENTS

Welcome

I am very excited that you have decided to take charge of your health! Bringing awareness to where you are at physically, mentally, emotionally and spiritually will be an eye-opening experience and proven to make a difference in your health and in your life. The small changes, tweaks and improvements you make during the Refresh will add up to monumental results.

Stay true to the guidelines. And remember that you will get out of this exactly what you put into it. The key to success is planning ahead! My 'preparation week' will give you time to shop and prepare yourself.

Now…take a moment to ask yourself "How am I?"

Most of us don't even think before we answer "I'm fine, thanks." But *really* take a moment, right now.

Close your eyes and ask yourself how you are.

Are you nervous? Content? Happy? Tired? Constipated?

Getting used to noticing ourselves and being aware of how we feel is the first step towards true health.

If you take away nothing else from the Refresh, I hope that you become more mindful of your body and its feelings. You will go through many states of 'being' during the three weeks. You might be anxious to get started. And then after three days, you might wonder why you're even doing this! Or you might feel energized and alert for the first time in a while! It is all part of the journey.

They say that 21 days is the average amount of time it takes someone to break a habit. I don't want to give you the impression that good health can be achieved instantly either. To make real, lasting changes in your body, you need to change your diet and lifestyle for more than three weeks! This is just the beginning...

My intention is that you experiment, explore and engage yourself in this whole process. The Attain True Health Body and Mind Refresh is designed to help you bring awareness to your body, diet and lifestyle choices. You will most likely gain a deeper understanding of what works best for your own body.

One person may find themselves with increased energy and focus, another may find they are less congested and yet another person's skin might clear up. Everyone is different and your experience will be different.

It might be very difficult for some because you have to give up some of your 'favorites'. But try and stick with it. If you attempt to try new foods and cook meals you would never have attempted before, you might be pleasantly surprised at how easy it is and how good it tastes. Eventually your body might not even want some of the old foods you were used to. And when you start noticing that you have more energy, your aches and pains have gone away and you can think more clearly, then you will know it's really worth it!

Remember...eat real, live mindfully, laugh often!

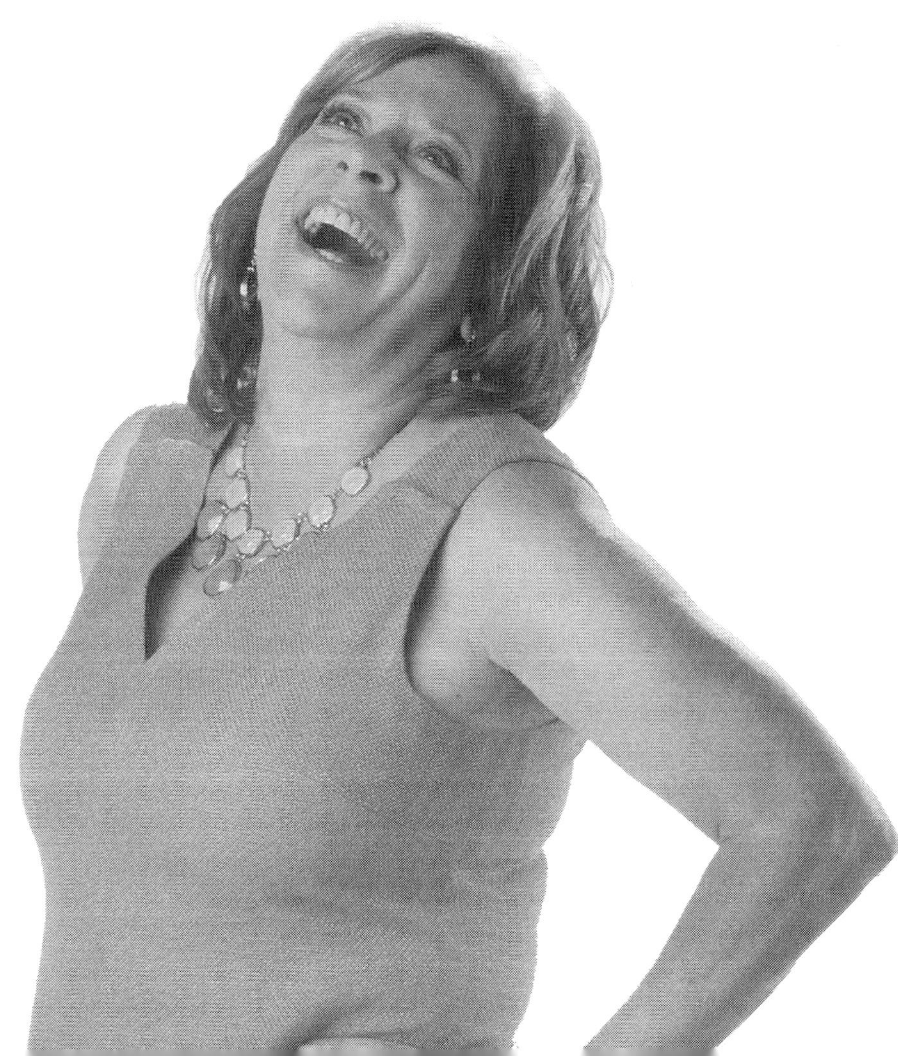

Getting Started

Fatigue, low energy, brain fog, excess weight...

These are only a few of the symptoms that affect our body when we are out of balance.

Just as our computer gets 'tired' and slows down when it is doing certain tasks and running programs over a long period of time, once refreshed, it becomes more active.

A Refresh means to give new strength or energy; to reinvigorate.

IS IT TIME TO REFRESH YOUR BODY?

A body in balance runs efficiently and effectively. When we are in balance we have energy and vitality. When we are out of balance we have "dis-ease" and inefficiency.

And there are many things that can throw the body out of balance, in fact it happens on a daily basis, sometimes minute to minute. Each day there are 'pebbles' that tilt our scale – eating processed foods, drinking too much alcohol, road rage, lack of sleep, unhappy relationships, stressful job and the list goes on. These particular daily circumstances can tilt the scale to one side or the other and if they happen continually, the scale (our body) stays askew.

And then there are the 'boulders', those big things that really knock us off our feet such as a divorce, the loss of a loved one or job. These can be traumatic and life changing. Our body senses when things are not right and tries very hard to keep itself in balance. But weighted down with physical and emotional pain from a life-changing event, the body might need some assistance.

I consider myself a pretty healthy person. But a few years ago I went through a divorce. Before it happened, I was healthy, happy, full of vigor, active, ate well, and took on each day like I was twenty years old. But in less than a year, my body started to break down.

I was worrying constantly about whether I could pay my bills. I wasn't being particularly healthy in the way I ate since it wasn't much fun to cook for one. I wasn't sleeping properly so I stopped meditating in order to sleep in. And I didn't have time to go to the gym and yoga classes because I found myself working up to sixteen hours a day to grow my Integrative Nutrition practice.

It all added up and my body became inflamed.

I carried an extra twenty pounds around my middle and on my face. I noticed new wrinkles appearing. More importantly, I couldn't think straight because I was suffering from brain fog.

I needed to change my lifestyle.

I started include habits that allowed my body to naturally refresh and to detoxify itself.

It improved not only my appearance, but also my thinking, my energy and productivity, my weight, and my sleep. And, yes, it's improved my relationships, too!

Even if your life is stress free, even if you eat well, use non-toxic household cleaners and organic skin care, move your body daily, and practice meditation, research has shown you still probably need to tweak your scale because we are living in a toxic world. Our bodies need to continually maintain that balance in order to remain healthy and live longer.

Since the 1950's, there have been over 70,000 new toxins introduced into our environments. And The Environmental Working Group tested the blood and urine of people around the country and found the average person carries 92 toxins within their body. This means there are devastating effects of toxic exposure on the human body. Toxins weaken our body's ability to burn fat, weaken our immune system and cause disease.

Once I let my guard down, I started to feel the effects of a body that was not operating at peak.

Do you suffer from low energy, aches and pains, allergies, constipation, skin problems, difficulty getting up in the morning or inflammation? Or you have lost weight and gained it back over and over again? Then this proven Refresh might be just what you need!

As we enjoy and admire the comforts of our modern life we sometimes fail to realize the onslaught of chemicals, toxins and processing procedures that have made our food supply, environment and beauty products silent killers. And the effect our words, thoughts, and behaviors have on our mental well-being.

The Refresh opened my eyes to a health connection. Several years ago, I began experiencing extreme blood sugar lows—and in tests my glucose level dropped to 30. Just a year or so later, I was diagnosed with Hashimoto's/Thyroiditis and given medication. My extreme sugar lows continued, even though I incorporated more protein into my meals, and ate more frequently in snack-sized portions. The Refresh inspired me to eliminate gluten, as I learned there might be a connection between celiac/gluten-intolerance and Hashimoto's. Since Refreshing and being gluten-free, I have not had a sugar crash. I feel positive and rejuvenated. The Refresh was the start of it all.

–Michele M.

Due to this onslaught, it is unfortunate that:

- The air we breathe is toxic with carbon monoxide, lead, mercury, radon, formaldehyde, benzene, nitric and sulfur oxides.
- Our water is contaminated from pesticides, herbicides, and fertilizers.
- Our food supply is bombarded with steroids, antibiotics, pesticides, hormones, dyes and waxes that are used in and on our food.
- There are dangerous chemicals found in personal care products such as parabens, phthalates, sodium lauryl sulfate and fluoride.
- The prescription drugs and over-the-counter medications have so many side effects that they actually do more harm than good.

It really is no wonder that our bodies are sometimes out of balance!

Here is a list of some of the diseases that are often directly linked to a buildup of toxins:

Psoriasis	Rheumatoid Arthritis	Lupus
Cancer	Fatigue	Fibromyalgia
Depression	Mental illness	Diabetes
Insomnia	Crohn's Disease	Hypertension
Obesity	Multiple Sclerosis	Memory loss
Ulcerative Colitis	Menstrual problems	Asthma
Abdominal bloating	Irritable Bowel Syndrome	

So what does this all mean? It means it can be hard to stay healthy in today's world! The good news is that your body is designed to filter toxins from our food and environment. While it is virtually impossible to avoid toxins on a day to day basis, it is possible, and even relatively easy, to reduce your exposure, giving your body a much needed rest.

My Attain True Health Body and Mind Refresh can play a significant part in achieving and maintaining optimum health and overcoming long standing health problems.

It is an effective way to assist you in achieving a healthy, vibrant body.

Over the course of 21 days, we will gently refresh our physical body, our emotional well-being, and our spiritual center.

The benefits of the Attain True Health Body and Mind Refresh include:

* Getting rid of toxic build-up
* Jumpstarting your weight loss
* Resetting the body's metabolism
* Feeling lighter and reduce bloating
* Gaining Energy
* Boosting Your Immune System
* Lessening aches and pains
* Improving mental clarity
* Establishing balance

And so much more.... This book will allow you to Refresh a few times of year to keep your body and mind in optimal balance!

SO, HOW DOES IT WORK?

The program is designed in three parts, taking place over five weeks.

The first week will be the Preparation Week. You begin the reduction or elimination of the food items that tax our liver (see Foods to Avoid on page 20). We want to give our digestive system a rest during the Refresh. With less of a toxic load from the food items we eliminate, it can work more efficiently.

But there will be lots of Foods to Enjoy as you'll see on pages 29-31. This list will also help you begin your shopping list.

Take the short Toxicity and Inflammation Quiz at the back of this book starting on pages 241 and your Vital Statistics on page 250. We will do both of these at the conclusion of the Refresh as well so we can make a comparison.

Then order the supplements and protein powder that enhance your detoxification process (all that information is on page 252). And lastly, fill out the checklist on page 25 to make sure you have completed all your Prep Week assignments.

Beginning on page 37, the book is divided into three chapters that will guide you over the three Refresh weeks with instructions and lifestyle suggestions to enhance your program.

After your 21 days are complete, the Post Week Chapter on page 68 will show you how to ease yourself back into your normal, daily routine.

Suggestions for meal plans, recipes, and grocery lists, start on page 115.

HOW WILL I KNOW WHAT TO DO?

This book will be like having me by your side every step of the way and will provide you with the tools you need. You will have the complete guidelines outlined for you, as well as, daily inspirations and checklists to keep you on track.

Prep Week

Your first task during the Preparation Week is to set your intentions. So...

ASK YOURSELF THE FOLLOWING QUESTIONS:

1. Why are you participating in the Refresh?
2. What are you hoping to achieve?
3. What about your relationship with food are you ready to leave in the past?
4. What do you want to experience more of in your life? (e.g. energy, health, power, freedom, balance, self-esteem, confidence, etc.)

YOUR KEYS TO SUCCESS:

1. Know what you want to get out of the Refresh.
2. Know what is possible.
3. Know you deserve it!
4. Take actions (like the Refresh) that align with your intention.
5. Learn from those actions and set new goals for yourself, applying the lessons learned.

READY?..OK...
HERE ARE THE FOODS TO AVOID

This will be the hardest part of the Refresh but the most beneficial. Remember that the purpose here is to reduce or eliminate the items we consume that put a strain on our liver and our digestive system.

The foods that are addictive or difficult to digest are obviously going to be the hardest and take the most effort.

We will be adding in foods that help nourish those areas and detoxify us. But in order to reap the benefits of the Refresh we need to avoid the following as much as possible:

CAFFEINE

During the Prep Week, please try to reduce the amount of caffeine you consume each day. By the first week of the Refresh, it would be helpful if you have eliminated it all together, but I'll give you two weeks!

THE CAFFEINE WEAN:

If you are a coffee drinker, begin slowly weaning yourself off caffeine during this Prep Week by moving through the following sequence:

1. Less coffee—reduce your intake by a cup each day; if you drink more than 2 cups a day, reduce by half and go from there
2. By day 3 or 4 of the Prep Week, you should be down to 1 cup a day
3. Then go to half-caffeine and half decaffeinated
4. Then decaffeinated only
5. Now try black tea, no coffee
6. Then move towards herbal teas

Alternative choices: herbal teas, or decaf green tea. For those of you that really need that taste of coffee, there are two brands I recommend. Teaccino is an organic, herbal coffee, naturally caffeine-free made from carob, organic barley, organic chicory, and ramon nuts. The other is called Dandy Blend. A blend of water-soluble extracts of roasted roots of dandelion, chicory and beets, and the grains of barley and rye. (And yes it is gluten free even though it contains barley and rye grains. The process they use is explained on their website).

SUGAR

Sugar weakens the body, causes inflammation, lowers your immune system, causes fatigue, and is highly addictive. We want to eliminate all forms of processed sugar in order to free your body of this addictive substance and build your strength.

During the Prep Week, this is your opportunity to try some of the natural or alternative sweeteners on the market. I need you to become a label detective.

I'll give you a head start. Let's take a look at where sugar is hiding. Sugar can be found in ketchups, salad dressings and even baby foods. It shows up on ingredient lists as:

Agave syrup, aspartame, barley malt, beet sugar, cane sugar, cane syrup, confectioner's sugar, crystalline fructose, crystalline sugar, date sugar, evaporated cane sugar, fructose, glucose, galactose, glucose, granulated sugar, high fructose corn syrup, honey, invert sugar, lactose, maltose, maple syrup, molasses, raw sugar, rice syrup, saccharin, sucanat, sucralose, sugarcane syrup, table sugar, turbinado, white sugar.

Our body needs sugar for brain health and energy—specifically glucose. So while we are reducing the amounts of refined sugars you are getting during the Refresh, you won't fully eliminate all sugars during the program. You want to avoid all refined and artificial sugars, as well as sugar alcohols (sorbitol, mannitol, malitol, xylitol) and get your sweet fix through the more natural sugars such as raw agave, honey maple syrup and Stevia.

Also, please eliminate all simple, refined carbohydrates which include white bread, white flour, white rice, white

Alyson's guided Refresh is a very impressive program to experience. It's easy to follow and understand, reasonable, and thorough. The changes made through the experience are easily transferred into long-term habits and those of us who have participated are better for it! For me, my positive experiences include the following: my arthritis inflammation is way down, my quality of sleep is up, and my level of concentration in general is up. My overall desire for refined sugar is essentially non-existent and I've even lost some weight. Love it!

–Kristin C.

pasta, cookies, candy, donuts, cake, pastries, soda etc.

Alternative choices in moderation: honey, maple syrup, brown rice syrup, molasses, raw agave nectar, raw coconut nectar, organic coconut palm sugar or Stevia (not Truvia!)

One teaspoon of sugar is equal to 4 grams. Just as an example – a 20 oz. bottle of cola has 16 teaspoons of sugar.

DAIRY

I am not of the opinion that dairy is necessarily bad for you. However, milk products create mucus in the body and are difficult to digest. Many people are allergic and/or lack the necessary enzymes to properly digest dairy. For the purpose of the Refresh, we will be giving up cow's milk dairy since that is the most allergenic. If at all possible, please try to avoid dairy in general. But if you need to have an occasional yogurt or cheese, goat or sheep varieties are best.

Eggs are not considered dairy since they come from a chicken, not a cow. Although many people do have egg sensitivities, we will keep eggs as one of our protein sources. Please buy only high quality, organic, free-range eggs.

Alternative choices: non-dairy milks, yogurts and cheeses made from coconut milk, almond milk, non-GMO soy, rice, hemp, cashew, flax etc.

MEAT

Simply put, meat is very hard to digest. So in order to give your system a break, it is advisable to eliminate red meat and pork from your diet during the Prep Week. An occasional 4 oz. piece of chicken or fish is okay if you are involved in a lot of physical activity or you feel weak. But everyone's body is different so please pay attention to how you feel. I feel it is important to have some type of protein at every meal. Therefore, we will be adding in a protein shake each day using the Shaklee Life protein powder. (Refer to the Product Ordering page for ordering information.) And you will be expected to have a source of protein at lunch and dinner as well.

Alternative choices: poultry, seafood, beans,, eggs, non-GMO soy products (such as tofu, tempeh), nuts, seeds, protein powders and quinoa.

ALCOHOL

Alcohol is a depressant, dehydrates your body and strains your liver. Enough said. If you want the body to run at optimal levels, alcohol has to go for 21 days!

WHEAT

Many people are unaware of their wheat (gluten) allergy because symptoms can come in many forms - from bloating to eczema to itchy eyes. In addition, the complex structure of wheat is relatively difficult to digest. By eliminating wheat (gluten) for this short period of time, you may notice a big difference in how your body feels. After all, isn't what this is all about? I will include recipes starting in Week One that contain gluten-free grains such as buckwheat quinoa, amaranth, millet, teff etc.

Take a moment to take a deep breath and acknowledge yourself for doing this Refresh. By removing these foods out of your life for 21 days, you will experience extraordinary benefits for your body,

The six main food items on the previous pages that we are avoiding are on the list because they are either addictive (sugar, caffeine, alcohol), allergenic (dairy and gluten), hard to digest (red meat and pork) or acidic (all of them).

This is also a time to stop putting more 'toxins' into the body in order to allow our elimination organs to do their job and get rid of 'old' toxic waste. Since many of the foods we eat today contain preservatives, additives, dyes and many other forms of toxins, the more we avoid these during the Refresh, the more time our elimination organs have to get rid of old waste that has been there for years! Therefore, in order to truly reap the benefits of this Refresh, I will take this opportunity to list a few other (somewhat obvious) items that should be avoided:

TOBACCO

If you smoke, I am sure it would be difficult to add this to your list of things to avoid. However, this might just be the opportunity you were looking for to either stop or cut back on cigarettes.

PROCESSED FOODS

Anything that comes in a box has been at least somewhat processed. As tasty as Paul Newman-O's are, a cookie is a cookie, no matter how you package it. Yes, organic ingredients are better for you. But organic cookies are still heavily processed and filled with fat and sugar, which your body metabolizes the same way it does the original kinds. So, just be aware that we are trying to eat real foods that don't come out of a box (so we do not take in any more toxins during the 21 days). I understand that we are all busy but do the best you can to avoid foods that are processed in any way. Real is the deal!

STIMULANTS

This includes decongestants, diet pills, ephedra and yerba matte. With the reduction of caffeine, you do not want to add any more stimulants into your diet during the Refresh.

ANIMAL FATS

Although I am allowing poultry (chicken, turkey, duck) during the Refresh as an added source of protein, it should be in moderation. I advise eating as little animal fat as possible during the 21 days. Try to find your protein in other healthier sources. That also means to reduce your intake of butter. It is allowed, but in moderation. And please remember that although chicken and turkey are allowed, it is advisable to not eat them as cold cuts. Cold cuts are processed meat that contain preservatives, additives, sodium nitrate and other toxins.

ALL WHITE FLOUR PRODUCTS

Obvious, but please read the labels on bread, crackers, rice cakes etc. Try to stick to whole grain or gluten free.

REFINED OILS AND HYDROGENATED FATS

Try to use only organic oils, preferably extra virgin olive oil and coconut oils for cooking and salads. Read the brands you have on hand and try to avoid:

a) Blended Vegetable Oils - Most commercial vegetable oils are a mixture of unidentified oils that have been extracted with chemicals.

b) Old Oils - Most oils have a limited shelf life, certainly no more than a year. Smell your oils. If they don't smell fresh, out they go. Rancid oils are hardly healthy.

c) Vegetable Shortenings - Usually made with partially

hydrogenated oils, shortenings are high in trans fats, which are considered the unhealthiest of all fats.

d) Chemically Extracted Oils - Although these are not proven to be dangerous, there are more natural methods of extraction, like cold pressing.

e) Oils High in Polyunsaturates - These include corn oil and soybean oil, among others. Polyunsaturates are not inherently unhealthy, but they do contain high levels of omega-6 fatty acids, which most Americans already get too much of. Although we need them in our diets, we should be getting fewer omega-6s and more omega-3s. The omega 3's can be found in flaxseed oil and walnut oil.

Please NOTE: Medications and/or Supplements
I am not a Medical Doctor. I DO NOT suggest that you eliminate any medications that you are presently taking for your health. If you are presently taking any vitamins and supplements other than the ones I am recommending, I would suggest stopping those during the Refresh. The supplements I am recommending contain only natural ingredients and will not conflict with any medication except if you are on a blood thinner (coumadin), I do not recommend any Vitamin K.

BUT NOW…FOODS TO ENJOY!

VEGETABLES

Arugula, Asparagus, Beets, Bok Choy, Broccoli, Broccoli Rab, Brussels Sprouts, Cabbage, Carrots, Cauliflower, Dandelion Greens, Green Beans, Kale, Kohlrabi, Leeks, Mushrooms, Onions, Peas, Radishes, Spinach, Summer, Squash, Sweet Potatoes, Swiss Chard, Tomatoes, Watercress, Zucchini.

FRUITS

Apples, Apricot, Avocado, Banana, Blackberries, Blueberries, Cantaloupe, Cherries, Clementine, Coconut, Dates, Figs, Grapefruit, Guava, Kiwi, Mango, Nectarine, Orange, Papaya, Peach, Pear, Pineapple, Pomegranate, Raspberries, Strawberries, Watermelon.

NUTS AND SEEDS

Almonds, Cashews, Flax Seeds Hazelnuts, Nut Butters, Peanuts, Pistachios, Pumpkin Seeds, Sesame Seeds, Sunflower Seeds, Walnuts.

HEALTHY FATS

Extra Virgin Olive Oil, Flax Seed Oil, Olive Oil, Sesame Oil, Virgin Coconut Oil.

GRAINS

Amaranth, Brown Rice, Buckwheat, Corn, Millet, Oats (GF variety), Quinoa, Rice, Teff.

The Foods to Enjoy list is by no means a complete list. I have included the fruits and vegetables that are seasonal and can easily be found in grocery stores or at Farmer's Markets. Remember to eat for the season, local whenever possible! And please try new things.

You can also have breads if they are made with gluten free grains and condiments such as peanut butter if it is organic and contains only peanuts and no sugar (my favorite brand is Woodstock Farms, Easy Spread), Vegenaise instead of regular mayonnaise since it contains no dairy (my favorite brand is Follow Your Heart), pastas – preferably made with gluten free grains. My favorite brands are Tinkyada and BioNaturea.

Fish choices should include cold-water fish such as wild salmon, cod, halibut, tilapia, sole, sardines, herring, mackerel. And your chicken should always be organic.

Obviously, if you already know that you have a hard time digesting or are allergic to certain fruits, vegetables, nuts or seeds, please continue to eliminate them from your diet. That probably goes without saying, but just in case.

Beneficial Beverages: Water and herbal teas are the beverages of choice during the Refresh. Add lemons/ limes or fruit concentrates to your water or plain, no sodium seltzer to make it interesting.

Here are a few suggestions for detoxifying teas:

a) Burdock Root–since it's a root, very grounding, also used for chronic skin disorders such as eczema and acne, boils and lung ailments.

b) Chamomile–gentle liver cleanser.

c) Fenugreek–helps to soften, dispel and dissolve mucus, making it good for the lungs and intestinal tract. Also helps regulate blood sugar levels.

d) Milk Thistle–protects the liver from free radical damage.

e) Peppermint–freshens breath and body odor during a cleanse and is stimulating. Make it extra strong to relieve headaches and sinus pressure.

f) Tulsi–a stimulating drink that helps you beat stress and fight free radicals. Other benefits – it helps boost stamina, increases energy and supports overall wellbeing.

GROCERY STAPLE LIST

You might want to stock your pantry with some of the following items prior to the beginning of the Refresh.

These are the recommended staples. You can decide what you will actually need depending upon what your menu choices are. Menus start on page 116.

Your Favorite Fresh Vegetables–a variety
Your Favorite Fresh Fruits–a variety
Dried Lentils or Beans of your choice
Canned Beans of your choice
Vegetable or Chicken Broths
Raisins and/or Prunes
Nuts–walnuts, almonds, pine nuts or any of your favorites
Extra Virgin Olive Oil and Extra Virgin Coconut Oil
Bragg's Apple Cider Vinegar
Balsamic Vinegar, Rice Wine Vinegar or some other vinegars of your choice for dressings
Ground Flaxseed (or you can buy the whole flaxseeds and grind them yourself)
Sea Salt–good quality
Condiments–such as mirin, miso, tahini (we will use these in many recipes)
Lemons
Fresh Ginger
Fresh Garlic
Fresh Herbs–Basil, Cilantro, Dill, Mint

Spices–check your pantry to see what spices you already have. The following list is a few of the spices we will be using in many of the recipes. These are helpful for reducing inflammation and detoxifying you:

Cinnamon, Chili Powder, Cloves, Cumin, Curry, Ginger, Ground Black Pepper, Oregano, Red Chili Flakes

Protein Powder–no whey. Instructions on ordering your protein powder for your morning smoothies are on page 130.

Gluten Free Grains–Please visit the bulk section of any health food store and buy a variety in small quantities so that you can sample them all.

IMPORTANT TO NOTE NOW:

Basically, once the Refresh begins this is what needs to be done on a daily basis. More details on the following are on page 38.

1. Upon waking, drink a cup of hot water with the juice of 1/2 lemon to wake up the liver.

2. Eat plenty of fresh fruit, vegetables, seeds, nuts, legumes and healthy fats.

3. Emphasize dark, leafy greens.

4. To satisfy protein requirements, chicken, and fish, as well as protein drinks are allowed.

5. Eat whole, intact gluten free grains.

6. Drink water, water, water.

7. Add flaxseed and apple cider vinegar to your meals every day.

8. Stick to only real food, nothing boxed, processed or 'fast'.

CHECK LIST FOR PREP WEEK

Make sure you have read up to this page really carefully so you truly understand the program. If you have any doubts, take your time to read it again. Then... order your protein powder and supplements (page 252) so they will arrive by Week One. Now tick off the following items as you complete them.

Set my intention.

____

____

____

____

____

_____ Take the Toxicity and Inflammation Quiz (page 241)

_____ Take my vital statistics.

Slowly reduce caffeine intake. How am I going to do that?
1. ______________________________
2. ______________________________
3. ______________________________

Slowly reduce sugar intake. How am I going to do that?
1.______________________________
2.______________________________
3.______________________________

_____ Eliminate red meat and pork.

_____Eliminate dairy products including milk, yogurt, and cheese.

Slowly reduce alcohol intake. How am I going to do that?

1.____

2.____

_____ Shop for the grocery staples for my pantry

Week One

Now you're ready to really get into your Refresh!

You will continue to reduce and eliminate sugar, caffeine, meat, dairy, gluten and alcohol that you started to cut back on during the prep week. Hopefully, by the end of this week you should be pretty much done with all of them. (Remember, it's only a few weeks and your body will thank you!)

This week we begin by adding in fabulous, real, fresh food, just the way Mother Nature intended. If you don't cook a lot or are not that good in the kitchen, I hope you are pleasantly surprised by what little effort it takes to make delicious, nutritious food for you and your family.

In order to stay on track, I have included a daily inspiration for you to follow and a place to journal your thoughts. Please go to the Keeping Track section each day starting on page 75.

HERE ARE THE BASIC REFRESH GUIDELINES AGAIN:

Do the best you can! If one day you get stuck in the mall and you are starving for lunch—that's OK. Look for a decent meal option that fits the plan, but if not, don't sweat it too much. There is no one watching over you; you are doing this for yourself. What you put in, you will get out. Even if you follow these guidelines half of the time, you will be doing your body a huge favor.

1. DRINK A CUP OF WARM WATER AND THE JUICE OF ONE-QUARTER OF A LEMON UPON WAKING EACH MORNING.

Warm water with lemon is the perfect wake up call for your digestive system. And it supports elimination so it is perfect for those with constipation problems. Lemon also purifies the blood and supports the immune system. A perfect detoxifier!

2. EAT PLENTY OF FRESH FRUITS, VEGETABLES, BEANS, NUTS, SEEDS AND YES, FATS!

This is the mainstay of your diet (plus the gluten free grains and your protein) over the next three weeks. Mix it up, experiment, explore and try things you wouldn't have dared before. Find five things listed here you have never tried and put them on your grocery list for this week.

Fruits, vegetables, nuts, seeds and legumes are complex carbohydrates. Over 50% of your daily food intake should come from complex carbs. When people say they are going on a low-carb diet, what they should say is they are going to cut out the refined, simple carbs such as white breads, pastas, white rice and white sugar.

For purposes of this Refresh we are basically on a complex carb diet for 3 weeks. You can eat all the complex carbs you want during the next three weeks!

Fruits

You should begin your day with fruit. After your cup of hot water and lemon you should either have a morning smoothie with some added fruit (see recipe section) or if you have chosen to have breakfast also, please add in some fruit with your eggs etc. Either way, start your day with fruit. Fruit is the fastest food to digest and is easily assimilated.

And you may have a piece of fruit as a snack mid-morning or afternoon, as well as incorporating some fresh fruit into your meal planning each day. Some fruits won't last as long as others, so plan accordingly. Buy lots of fresh berries such as strawberries, blueberries, raspberries, and blackberries and eat them up within the first few days. Remember what I said about having to go to the grocery store at least twice a week!

Other fruits such as apples, oranges, pears, and the fruits with thick skins such as cantaloupe, honeydew, watermelon, mango, papaya, etc. will last longer. Enjoy! Fruit could be the answer to your sugar cravings too! (See my information on organic vs. non-organic on page 128.)

Vegetables

So many choices, so little time! I love vegetables!

During the Refresh, you should try to eat as many vegetables as possible at every meal of the day. Sautéed, stewed, baked, roasted, chopped, diced, julienned and even raw! Here's your chance to experiment, explore and learn. Think outside the box, try new ones and freshen up your old standbys. Utilize the many recipes I have provided and dig out your old cookbooks.

Nuts and Seeds.

Full of healthy fats and tons of fiber! Try to buy raw, organic and unsalted, if possible. Keep nuts and seeds in the refrigerator because they have essential oils that go rancid very quickly. Soaking nuts and seeds overnight will make them easier to digest. And it is important to chew them very well so they don't pass through your digestive system whole.

Use the health food store to buy a variety of nuts in small quantities. That way you won't spend a lot of money and you have the opportunity to see if you enjoy them.

Beans and Legumes

These are one of your major sources of protein on the Refresh. Try to eat at least one serving every day. Small beans are easier to digest than larger beans. Either canned or dried is fine, but look for the organic, BPA (bisphenol-A) free cans. My top four favorite companies that use this type of toxin-free lining include Eden, Trader Joe's, Native Forest and Vital Choice. Dried beans cook faster if you soak them overnight. And if using canned, please rinse them to get any sodium off. Beans and legumes are full of fiber and that allows the natural sugars to absorb slowly into your bloodstream, not causing spikes. Plus they are very filling and quite tasty! Experiment!

Healthy Fats

Yes, eat healthy fats such as extra virgin olive oil for dressings and light sautés, regular olive oil for roasting vegetables at higher temperatures, sesame oil for stir-frys and dressings, coconut oil for sautéing and protein drinks and flaxseed oil for dressings and proteins drinks too.

NOTE: Flaxseed oil cannot be used to cook with. It is best to use as part of your oil in a salad dressing (e.g. if the recipe calls for one cup of oil – use 1/4 cup of flaxseed and 3⁄4 cup of extra virgin olive oil. That way you get even more essential fatty acids into your daily diet. And flaxseed oil needs to be stored in the refrigerator).

3. EMPHASIZE DARK, GREEN LEAFY VEGETABLES (AT LEAST ONE SERVING A DAY).

Do you know what the #1 vegetable in the American diet is? Potatoes! And usually served as French fries! Not to knock the potato, but there are so many wonderful vegetables out there to fill our plates with during the Refresh that give us way more nourishment and energy than French fries ever could.

Focus on dark, green, leafy vegetables (at least one serving a day during the Refresh, preferably more). Now is the time to discover all the tasty and healthy ways you can prepare them and that doesn't mean boiling them until they turn gray! Greens are full of vitamins, folic acid and calcium. You can get more calcium for your bones from eating kale than you can from a glass of milk! The leaves also contain chlorophyll which is absorbed from the sun's energy. By eating greens, that energy is transferred to you.

Greens strengthen our immune system, improve liver, kidney and gall bladder function, fight depression, clear congestion, improve circulation and keep our skin clear. Wow!

And don't forget the cruciferae family. Some of my favorite cruciferous vegetables include Brussels sprouts, cabbage, broccoli, broccoli rabe, kohlrabi, cauliflower, bok choy, kale, watercress and arugula. Cruciferous vegetables contain phytonutrients that increase production of enzymes involved in detoxification. The result? Our cells are able to clear free radicals and toxins, including potential carcinogens, lowering our risk of cancer. Another Wow! One serving a day (preferably much more!)

Some examples of Dark Leafy Greens include:

- Arugula
- Beet Greens
- Bok Choy
- Chicory
- Collard Greens
- Dandelion Greens
- Escarole
- Kale – Curly, Dinosaur or Tuscan
- Lettuce – Any except Iceberg!
- Mustard Greens
- Spinach
- Swiss Chard
- Turnip Greens
- Watercress

4. EAT WHOLE, INTACT GLUTEN FREE GRAINS.

What does that mean? Whole grains contain all three parts of their natural structure—the bran, the germ and the endosperm. They are high in fiber and nutrients, unlike refined grains that are mostly simple carbohydrates. Refined grains retain only the endosperm. Keeping grains intact slows and prevents the digestion of starch and is responsible for preventing spikes in blood sugar. Try the many varieties of gluten free grains found in the bulk section of the health food store.

There are ten here – try some new ones:

- Amaranth
- Brown Rice
- Buckwheat
- Corn
- Millet
- Oats (gluten free variety)
- Quinoa (high in protein, contains all nine essential amino acids)
- Sorghum
- Teff
- Wild Rice

5. DRINK A LOT OF WATER!

H20 is the way to go... Ever try washing your car with soda? How about juice? Most bottled drinks are incredibly high in sugar and chemicals – not so great for cleaning. During the Refresh, substitute water for most of your other beverages so your body can Refresh itself effectively.

How much water? Everyone is different, but I know you need more than you have been drinking up until now. Start increasing your amount each day so by Week 2 you are up

Goodbye Aches and Pains, Sinus Headaches, Tingling Fingers, Constipation, Indigestion! Hello to Good Health and Physical Comfort! The Attain True Health Body and Mind Refresh has had such a major and positive impact on my life. I have become more attuned to my body and all of my regular negative symptoms have disappeared! In looking back at the experience, I realize that I had myself worked up about doing without. By the end of the second week, the physical changes and loss of uncomfortable symptoms took precedence and my mindset changed. I was able to appreciate feeling physically and mentally renewed. I am looking forward to doing it again in a few months!

Judy B.

to drinking half your body weight in ounces (i.e. if you weigh 150 pounds, drink 75 oz. of water per day – at least!). A good way to check if you have had enough is to look at the color of your urine. It should be the color of light straw, almost clear, every day.

Tired of plain water? Every animal on earth drinks water and nothing but water. Your body is made up of 75% water and so is the earth. Still tired of plain water?

Here are some ideas to try:

Seltzer (no sodium) or sparkling water

Add: lemon slices, lime slices, orange slices, cucumber slices, a splash of juice, mint or other fresh herbs, fresh ginger, a drop of flavored essential oils or extract

Fresh brewed ice tea made with herbal teas

Hot herbal teas

Pure coconut water (only ingredient should be unsweetened coconut water)

Juices made with all natural ingredients (no added sugars)

Aloe juice or POM pomegranate juice

Fruit juice concentrates – add a little to your water or seltzer to flavor it

6. GET YOUR PROTEIN REQUIREMENTS FROM BOTH YOUR MORNING SMOOTHIE AND OTHER SOURCES BESIDES RED MEAT OR PORK.

You will get 24 grams of protein in your morning smoothie. You can also have a smoothie for lunch or dinner if you choose since protein is satisfying and filling. But because red meat and pork are the two hardest foods to digest, I prefer that you eliminate them all together during the Refresh. You may occasionally have chicken or fish for your protein requirements. Some other recommended protein sources include:

Yogurt—made from goat's or sheep milk or a non-dairy variety made from coconut, almonds, rice, or non-GMO soy (found at the health food store)

Cheese—goat cheese and feta cheese in moderation and non-dairy varieties

Soy—please only buy organic and non-GMO (non-genetically modified) brands of soy products. My favorite soybean product is frozen edamame and non-GMO brand for tofu is Nasoya. Fermented soy products are preferred such as miso, tempeh, natto, kimchi and soy sauce.

Protein Powders—my recommendation for protein powder is the Shaklee Life Energizing Shake. I do not recommend any other brand during this Refresh since this is a proven and tested source. Please see page 252 for product ordering

Grains – quinoa, amaranth, brown rice, non-GMO corn, teff, buckwheat and millet contain protein and essential amino acids

Nuts and Seeds – enjoy them all for the protein and the fiber

Legumes – lentils, peas, beans, peanuts

7. ELIMINATE CAFFEINE, SUGAR, DAIRY, MEAT, GLUTEN AND ALCOHOL. See Prep Week information.

8. ADD GROUND FLAXSEED & APPLE CIDER VINEGAR INTO YOUR DAILY MEAL PLANNING

This is a very IMPORTANT part of the Attain True Health Body and Mind Refresh! In addition to eating clean, whole foods during the Refresh, the addition of ground flaxseed and apple cider vinegar will kick start your body into cleansing mode. Regardless of your meals, these can be added into your routine at any point during the day.

Ground Flaxseed: Each day, use 1 tablespoon (or more)

of ground flaxseed. Add it to your smoothie, sprinkle it on your breakfast, shake it over a salad or mix it into a rice bowl. Buy whole flaxseeds and grind only the amount you need to use each day. Or buy ground flaxseed or flax meal. It should be kept in the refrigerator to prevent it from turning rancid.

Bragg's Apple Cider Vinegar: Each day, drink 1 tablespoon in a small glass of water. Bragg's is raw, unfiltered vinegar that you can find at most grocery or health food stores. Please buy the Bragg's brand. It is organic and alkalizing. I rely on Bragg's to clear congestion and help digestion. According to Bragg's website, benefits are:

Rich in enzymes and potassium
Supports a healthy immune system
Promotes digestion and pH balance
Helps sooth sore throats
Helps remove body sludge and toxins
Helps maintain healthy skin
Helps promote youthful, healthy bodies

9. REDUCE OR ELIMINATE ALL FOODS THAT ARE PROCESSED, BOXED OR 'FAST'. Self-explanatory!

10. STICK TO REAL FOOD!

This may be the simplest and most important piece of the whole Refresh! It doesn't matter if you eat spinach or kale, black beans or kidney beans, almonds or walnuts. The point is – these are all real food.

So what's not real food? Things like frozen dinners, boxed lunches or mac and cheese, Doritos. You may be able to find a packaged product that has no sugar, caffeine, dairy, gluten or meat – but that doesn't mean it's healthy!

Is it REAL food?

Answer 'yes' to these questions:

Does it have fewer than 5 ingredients?

Can I pronounce all the ingredients?

Would my great grandmother recognize it as food?

Is it possible to grow this in the ground or make it in the average kitchen?

Week Two

Hooray! You've made it to Week Two.

The hard part is over. By now you should have totally eliminated sugar, caffeine, dairy, meat, gluten and alcohol. And we are not adding anything new to the 'eliminate' list during this week. In the next seven days you will begin to incorporate simple lifestyle suggestions to optimize your body's ability to detoxify itself.

During Week Two you'll continue the same basic guidelines as Week One. See the chart again on page 27.

But now we're going to add in some simple routines for you to follow

1. Allow detoxification time before bed
2. Practice movement and deep breathing
3. Evaluate personal care products
4. Exfoliate dead skin
5. Learn ways to de-stress

Here they are in detail:

1. ALLOW TIME FOR DETOXIFICATION BEFORE BED.

One of the reasons our bodies become sluggish is because our system is overworked. With the amount of toxins we normally surround ourselves with each day, through no fault of our own most of the time, our elimination systems are on overtime.

What would happen if you worked all the time at your job with no breaks? Well, for starters, your desk would be a mess, not to mention the rest of your life. And you would be exhausted. Just like you, your digestive system needs a break. When it is supposed to be digesting food, it can't clean house. So during Week Two, we want to help our body detoxify naturally by giving our systems some down time. You have been very effective by eliminating some of the items that tax the system such as sugar, caffeine, dairy, meat, gluten and alcohol. So the next step is to let it do its job!

Leave Two Hours Between your Last Meal and Bedtime!

At the office or school, there is a janitorial staff that cleans overnight. Your body works like that too. Don't let a late night dinner or snack get in the way of overnight cleaning. To help your body do its job, leave at least two hours between your last meal and bedtime.

And Consider This:

When our meals are nutrient-poor, we hunger for something more. When our meals are full of sugar or too many simple carbohydrates that turn to sugar quickly (like fast food or processed food) our blood sugar spikes, then falls, and leaves us feeling starved for more.

My advice is not to eat all day long to try to feel satisfied; the human body was not designed to eat all day long. Our hunter and gatherer ancestors did not have the luxury of a Starbucks on every corner to satisfy their coffee or scone craving between meals. The truth is, if you eat whole, real, nutrient-dense foods, 3 meals a day should be enough. I'm not saying you should never snack, but notice over the next week if you increase your portion sizes of real food, whether or not you actually need that snack. Just eat, and eat well at mealtimes. Eat until you are satisfied. Eat a healthy dessert, if you choose. Then give your digestive system a rest for the night and let it do its job!

2. PRACTICE MOVEMENT AND DEEP BREATHING

Movement on the outside creates movement on the inside! Whether you are an avid gym goer or have never tied on a pair of running shoes in your life, movement this week is important. Movement will help massage your organs and help to stimulate them to do their job most efficiently while relieving stress. So during Week Two, I would suggest you practice some form of movement and deep breathing at least once a day.

Twist and Shout!

OK, you don't have to shout while doing this twisting exercise (but it actually can't hurt because pushing out the air from deep in your lugs is detoxifying, getting out the stale air that stays way down deep at the bottom of your lungs. See deep breathing below). These twists will relieve tension and aid digestion. Known as the Supine Spinal Twist or to my yogi friends, the Double Knee Down Twist:

Lie on your back, hug your knees to your chest

Open your arms out to either side forming a T shape

Allow your knees to slowly fall to the right side of your body; adjust for any back discomfort

Turn your head to the left. Relax and breathe.

Slowly bring your knees up and over, letting them fall to the left side

Turn your head to the right. Relax and breathe.

Repeat as often as you like!

Deep Breathing

As Americans, we tend to shallow breathe all day long. We rush around, not really conscious of how deep a breath we take. Your diaphragm muscle sits between your lungs and your digestive organs. While you inhale, it moves down and gently massages your belly organs. Often, we do not inhale fully into the belly from the shallow breathing we do. Instead of getting a gentle massage to our organs, we tend to take sort, quick huffs and puffs that could lead to anxiety, stress, depression and digestive trouble. So, during the Refresh (and hopefully much longer) try this breathing technique at night before bedtime:

Sit comfortably, on the floor or a chair, with a straight spine.

Place one hand on your belly.

Breathe normally, paying attention to each inhale and exhale.

Begin to slow and deepen your breath.

Try to complete what I call the '6-6-6 breath'.

Inhale deeply for 6 counts, hold for 6 counts, and exhale completely for 6 counts.

Notice your hand on your belly rise when you inhale. That means you are breathing down deep into your lungs and the diaphragm area.

Notice the feeling of your hand contracting when you exhale. Make sure you get all the air out of the bottom of your lungs.

Do this as many times as you like, listening to the silence and the sound of your own breathing.

3. EVALUATE PERSONAL CARE PRODUCTS

Your skin is the largest organ of your body and it absorbs up to 60% of what you put on it! And children absorb 40-50% more than adults. Reports state that one in eight of the 82,000 ingredients used in personal care products are industrial chemicals, including carcinogens, pesticides, reproductive toxins, and hormone disruptors. Many products include plasticizers (chemicals that keep concrete soft), degreasers (used to get grime off auto parts), and surfactants (they reduce surface tension in water, like in paint and inks). Imagine what that does to your skin and to the environment.

Did you realize that when you use common drug store shampoo to wash your hair, your liver is forced to process the same amount of nitrates you would get from eating an entire pound of bacon? And that's just from ONE shampooing!

Research discovered that the average woman is lathering her body in up to 515 different synthetic chemicals every day!!

Aside from perfume (which is responsible for about half the number of chemicals), an alarming amount of them are going directly on your face in the form of:

• foundation • concealer • powders • bronzer • blush • eyebrow pencils and powders • lipsticks and liners • eye liner • mascara • cleansers • moisturizers • exfoliation • make-up remover • eye cream • acne creams and lotions

A good rule of thumb is to only put on your skin what you would happily put in your mouth. How does that shampoo taste? How many pounds of lipstick do you eat a year? Sunblock for breakfast?

Of course, it is not really about how it tastes but rather what is in these products. Read labels for personal care products as carefully as you would your food labels because you are what you eat - and you are what you put on your skin. Women especially tend to be overexposed to toxins through our personal care products and makeup.

Here is a list of the most common toxins found in our skincare products:

1. BHA and BHT

BHA (butylated hydroxyanisole) and BHT (butylated hydroxytoluene) are used as preservatives in lipsticks and moisturizers, among other cosmetics. They interfere with hormone function, can induce allergic reactions in the skin and are known to cause liver, thyroid and kidney problems. They also affect lung function and blood coagulation. BHT can act as a tumor promoter in certain situations and could cause cancer.

2. Parabens

Parabens are widely used preservatives that prevent the growth of bacteria, mold and yeast in cosmetic products. Parabens possess estrogen-mimicking properties that are associated with increased risk of breast cancer in women, sterility in men, and early puberty in children. These are used in makeup, moisturizers, shampoos, deodorants etc. Look out for ingredients with "paraben" in their name (methylparaben, butylparaben, propylparaben, isobutylparaben, ethylparaben).

3. FD&C Color and Pigments

Synthetic colors from coal tar that contain heavy metal salts that deposit toxins in the skin, causing irritations. Absorption can cause depletion of oxygen, cancer and brain toxicity.

4. DEA, MEA and TEA

Commonly found in creamy and foaming products such as moisturizer and shampoo. Can react to form cancer-causing nitrosamines. Is a skin/eye irritant and causes dermatitis. Easily absorbed through the skin to accumulate in body organs and the brain.

5. Sodium Laureth Sulfate (SLES) and Sodium Lauryl Sulfate (SLS):

In products that foam such as shampoo, cleaners, bubble bath and also found in car washes, garage floor cleaners, engine degreasers and over 90% of our personal care products. Been known to cause cancer, damage our liver, depression, labored breathing, diarrhea and death.

6. Benzoyl Peroxide

Used in acne products. Possible tumor promoter. May act as a mutagen; produces DNA damage, is toxic when inhaled and is an eye, skin and respiratory irritant.

7. Phthalates

A group of chemicals used in hundreds of products to increase the flexibility and softness of plastics. The main phthalates in cosmetics and personal care products are dibutyl phthalate in nail polish, diethyl phthalate in perfumes and lotions, and dimethyl phthalate in hair spray. They are known to be endocrine disruptors and have been linked to increased risk of breast cancer, early breast development in girls, and reproductive birth defects in males and females. Unfortunately, it is not disclosed on every product as it's added to fragrances (remember the "secret formula" not listed); a major loophole in the law. They can be found in deodorants, perfumes/colognes, hair sprays and moisturizers.

8. Petroleum-Based Products

Toluene is a petrochemical derived from petroleum or coal tar sources. You may see it on labels listed as benzene, toluol, phenylmethane and methylbenzene. Toluene is a potent solvent able to dissolve paint and paint thinner. It can affect your respiratory system, cause nausea and irritate your skin. Expecting mothers should avoid exposure to toluene vapors as it may cause developmental damage in the fetus. Toluene has also been linked to immune system toxicity. It can be found in nail polish, nail treatments and hair color/bleaching products.

Check the safety of your products at: www.cosmeticsdatabase.com

This database was created by the Environmental Working Group (www.ewg.org)

I am not asking you to replace everything you use, but I am asking that you become aware of how much toxicity you are surrounded by in your home and what you are putting on your skin on a daily basis. During this Refresh, we are trying to reduce your toxic load, so maybe replacing a few items is a good idea. Being informed will simply allow you to make more intelligent and conscious choices for yourself, your family, and the planet as a whole. You might lose a couple of seconds of your life while looking for detrimental chemicals on product labels, but is that any match for the healthier years you'll add to your life, the illnesses you'll avoid, and the example you will be in support of a more sustainable world?

More information about the Shaklee Enfuselle products I recommend can be found at the end of this packet in the Product Ordering section on page 252.

4. DETOXIFY YOUR SKIN WITH EXFOLIATION

Skin grows from the inside out. Thus the skin cells on the outermost portion of your skin are usually dead and need sloughing off your body. During this time Refresh, there are many ways to help your skin eliminate toxins, one of them being a gentle brushing. A gentle brushing of the skin promotes better blood circulation, massages your lymph nodes (which are you waste/toxin transporters), and encourages cells to regenerate. The brushing can be done either dry or wet, it's your choice, but here are my recommendations:

Use a natural fiber bath brush (preferably with a long handle to help you reach hard-to-reach areas on your back) or a loofah.

For dry brushing: gently massage your skin with your loofah sponge or bath brush in small circular motions. You can start at your feet and move up towards your heart. Do the same thing with your arms starting from your hands and moving downward. Doing this dry will encourage blood circulation.

For wet brushing: after you're done washing up in the shower or bath, use the same technique as with dry brushing. (You can use an organic bath or shower gel to make the movement of your circular motions glide over your skin.) *It is important to squeeze your loofah sponge after use and to hang it so any excess moisture dries off.

5. LEARN WAYS TO DE-STRESS

Stress is a silent killer. It is also one of the leading causes of weight gain around the middle.

If we can find time throughout our day to de-stress, calm down and become centered, we would all feel so much better. Here are some tips for ways to de-stress:

Go for a Quick Walk.

Even if you can only spare five minutes, go for a walk, it might just be to the water cooler and back or it can be outside in Mother Nature. The aim here is to get yourself away from the immediate source of stress and to calm down. A few minutes to gather your thoughts is all you need to get some perspective.

Read Some Fiction.

If you're seriously worked up, upset or stressed, one of the best things to can do is grab a book. Fiction is ideal (especially anything funny or uplifting). Reading fiction takes you out of the here-and-now and into a different world. You can forget everything that's troubling you, for just ten minutes, as you concentrate on the story.

Meditate or Pray Often.

The best thing we can do to instantly de-stress is to simply stop everything. I always tell my clients about meditation. It really is quite simple, once you get the hang of it. Just sit up straight and try concentrating on your breath, just like in the deep breathing technique in #2 above. Some people believe they have to totally clear their mind and this takes a while to learn so perhaps concentrating on a calming image or a word or phrase is a good way to start. If your mind wanders, just bring it back. Eventually it will listen! Start out with only 5 minutes and see how it goes. If meditation isn't your thing yet, you can also pray – if this suits your religious/spiritual persuasions. It can be a very powerful way to get outside of your own head and call on a higher power for some much-needed help!

Watch a Funny Video.

I don't know about you, but I just can't stay stressed out when I'm laughing. Try watching 'Americas Funniest Home Videos' or your own home videos. Just give yourself five minutes to indulge. You'll find that you return to your work – or whatever the source of the stress is – feeling much better equipped to handle it.

Make an Herbal Tea.

A warm, soothing mug of herbal tea might do the trick. The act of stopping whatever it is that is stressing you gives you a chance to concentrate on something else. You'll probably also feel a psychological boost from doing something positive and nurturing for yourself.

Take a Warm Bath and use Aromatherapy

The recuperative and healing properties of water have many stress-relieving benefits. Submerging in a bath tub relieves your body from the constant pull of gravity, and heated water relaxes muscle tension, improving circulation, range of motion and energy flow. Melt away your stress by creating a mini spa in your bathroom. Turn on soothing music, dim the lights, light candles and prepare fresh towels. The music will drown out household sounds that you may associate with everyday stressors, and relaxed lighting can go a long way when creating a peaceful mood. You can pick up aromatherapy bubble bath, soap, skin- moisturizing oils and exfoliating body scrubs at your local store.

Take Slow, Deep Breaths.

When we get stressed, we tend to breathe more quickly, taking shallow breaths. (Some of us do this all day long, as part of our normal breathing!) Concentrate on your breathing (you might want to do this in conjunction with meditation or prayer). Imagine breathing from your stomach, not your chest. Take slow, deep, fulfilling breaths. Calming your body down physically in this way is likely to have a quite an effect on your frazzled mental state.

Week Three

Wow…Almost There! You made it to Week Three.

Congratulations!

Congratulations! You should be proud of yourself. I know this could have been a tough journey for you. There are many symptoms you could have experienced over the last two weeks such as hives, runny noses, headaches, gas pains, cramps, lack of bowel movements, fatigue, fogginess and even a flushed red face. And you might also have been in the kitchen cooking more often and introducing new foods to your family.

So with only one week to go, you might think that you can cheat a little because you are so close. But if you can keep it together for another seven days, your body will be thankful and I think you will see even more remarkable changes during this last week. Now that we have reduced our intake of toxins, the body has a chance to begin the 'cleaning out' process. It is imperative that you continue to drink lots of water to flush out those toxins that are on the move. Adding in movement, dry or wet brushing to the skin and ways to de- stress are also very beneficial to continue into Week Three.

The only addition this week is to try and introduce more raw and fermented foods. You have been eating a lot more salads, but eating even more raw vegetables and fruits will improve your digestion and increase the amounts of enzymes into your system that are normally killed by cooking.

Eating more fermented foods will also aid digestion, increase your good bacteria, up your enzyme intake and improve your immune system. Fermented foods have wonderful, natural 'live' cultures in them. These micro-organisms populate our digestive tract with beneficial gut flora. You have been germinating good bacteria since we started the Refresh by using the Shaklee Life Energizing

Shake which contains 1 billion colony-forming units of probiotics that are designed to make it thought the stomach acid and multiply and colonize in your gut! How exciting... by adding in even more foods that contain beneficial bacteria, your heath will improve greatly.

This week, continue your same morning routine with the lemon/water, flaxseed and vinegar, as well as your protein drink. And if you have been trying the variety of recipes I have provided in the Recipe section, please make sure to take a look this week for some new fun ideas with raw and fermented foods to try.

REFRESH GUIDELINES – WEEK THREE

Please remember that the guidelines for Weeks One and Two still apply during Week Three. There is only one addition this week: EXPERIMENT WITH RAW AND FERMENTED FOODS DAILY

What is raw food?

Living, raw, uncooked fruits, vegetables, nuts, seeds and sprouted grains/beans. You have actually already been incorporating most of this into your diet for the last two weeks. And you didn't even know you were becoming a raw foodist!

When food is cooked, the live enzymes are destroyed. Eating food that is alive means consuming more live enzymes —and that means your body has to do less work during digestion!

During Week Three, try experimenting by incorporating more raw foods into your daily diet in the form of salads, fresh fruit, green smoothies or any of the raw food recipes in the Recipe section provided. NOTE: If you are experiencing a lot of gas or pain with the raw foods, skip this and just try the fermented foods only.

TEN REASONS TO EAT MORE RAW FOODS

Live foods. It's common sense, right? A cooked seed won't grow, but a raw seed will. Heating food over 118 °F destroys much of the nutrients in your food. Cooking food also diminishes the natural life energy. We should all try to eat more uncooked food.

Enzymes. Cooking food destroys much of the natural enzymes (your body can also create enzymes, but can only do so much) in your food that are needed to break down nutrients. Eating raw eliminates this problem.

Energy. You won't know this unless you try it for yourself, but eating raw gives you an amazing boost in energy.

Better sleep and less sleep needed. You won't wake up feeling tired or groggy anymore. You'll wake up feeling full of energy.

Increased mental clarity. Eating raw with all its vitamins, enzymes and nutrients helps you focus better and might make you more emotionally in tune with yourself and others.

Eat as much as you want. This isn't really a health benefit, but it is pretty awesome. There aren't too many calories in raw vegetables, and they are nutrient-dense, so enjoy!

Less clean-up. Simply put, there aren't many dishes to wash when you eat fruit and vegetables. Although if you do compost, you'll probably have to do it more often.

No packaging. Eating raw means less packaging all around. This means less trash in a landfill and more room in your cupboards. Win/win for everyone.

More regularity. You should naturally have around two to three bowel movements a day. If you're going less than that, it probably means your intestines are unhealthily clogged. A raw diet gives you more than enough fiber to keep you regular.

Connection with the earth. Eating food that's been freshly picked just feels different. You feel more connected to the earth and more grounded. Eating lots of processed foods, frozen or from a box, creates more of a gap and leaves you feeling disconnected from the earth that sustains you.

What are fermented foods?

Fermented foods contain healthy forms of bacteria that aid digestion, relieve constipation, and help the body absorb vitamins and minerals. Our bodies are often depleted of healthy bacteria in our gut due to poor diets and use of antibiotics. Begin to replenish your intestinal flora by including fermented foods into your diet, such as pickles, sauerkraut, kimchee and miso. To get the most benefits from fermentation, you want to eat traditionally prepared foods; that means that standard deli pickles may not fit the bill.

In the past, fermentation was a common way of preparing food to enhance nutritional value and keep it from going bad in storage prior to the invention of refrigeration. It's very recent that fermented foods have begun to disappear from our plate. Modern pickles and sauerkraut are made with vinegar instead of the traditional method of lacto-fermentation using salt. Bread and pasta are made with commercial yeast instead of being naturally leavened with wild yeast (sourdough). Wine, beer and cheeses are being pasteurized — killing off all the good bacteria we so desperately need to maintain health.

But there are many advantages to going back to the traditional ways of our ancestors and eating more fermented foods. In the normal scheme of things, we'd never have to think twice about replenishing the bacteria that allow us to digest food. But since we're living with antibiotic drugs, chlorinated water, antibacterial soap and many other factors in our contemporary lives that I'd group together as a 'war on bacteria', we need to look at ways to replenish the good bacteria. If we fail, we won't effectively get nutrients out of the food we're eating.

Try some of the fermented food recipes in the recipe section, or go online and get even more recipes.

EIGHT REASONS TO EAT MORE FERMENTED FOODS

Fermented foods improve digestion. Fermenting our foods before we eat them is like partially digesting them before we consume them. According to Joanne Slavin, a professor in the Department of Food Science and Nutrition at the University of Minnesota, "...sometimes people who cannot tolerate milk can eat yogurt. That's because the lactose (which is usually the part people can't tolerate) in milk is broken down as the milk is fermented and turns into yogurt."

Fermented foods restore the proper balance of bacteria in the gut. Do you suffer from lactose intolerance? Gluten intolerance? Constipation? Irritable bowel syndrome? Yeast infections? Allergies? Asthma? All of these conditions have been linked to a lack of good bacteria in the gut.

Raw, fermented foods are rich in enzymes. Your body needs enzymes to properly digest, absorb, and make full use of your food. As you age, your body's supply of enzymes decreases. This has caused many scientists to hypothesize that if you could guard against enzyme depletion, you could live a longer, healthier life.

Fermenting food actually increases the vitamin content. According to the Nourished Kitchen blog, "Fermented dairy products consistently reveal an increased level of folic acid, as well as pyroxidine, B vitamins, riboflavin and biotin depending on the strains of bacteria present."

Eating fermented food helps us to absorb the nutrients we're consuming. You can ingest huge amounts of nutrients, but unless you actually absorb them, they're useless to you. When you improve digestion, you improve absorption.

Fermenting food helps to preserve it for longer periods of time. Milk will go bad in the fridge but kefir and yogurt last a lot longer. Sauerkraut pickles and salsa will keep for months. And if you've got a huge batch of produce in your garden that you don't know how to use up — ferment it!

Fermenting food is inexpensive. There's nothing fancy required for this hobby. And many of the foods required to make these recipes are very inexpensive. You can use inexpensive cabbage to make sauerkraut, or get yourself a kombucha scoby, and for 'just pennies', you've got a health elixir/soda.

Fermenting food increases the flavor. There's a reason humans enjoy drinking wine and eating stinky cheese. There's a reason we like sauerkraut on our hot dogs and salsa on our tortilla chips. It tastes good!

Information from from www.cheeseslave.com

Post Week

You Did It!

You have taken a huge step in the improvement of your overall health,

If you spoke with some of your friends during the Refresh weeks, they probably said "I could never give up all those things!" And maybe you were hesitant, prior to beginning, about whether or not you really could do it yourself. Whether you completed 3 days or 3 weeks, I hope that this experience has made a difference in your life. You are less toxic than when you started, that's for sure. But if you had other major improvements in your health, I would love for you to share them with all of us.

The Post Week Guidelines will give you some steps to take which ease you back in to mainstream living. My advice is to take it slow. Just like we had 7 days of Prep Week to try to ease into the elimination of sugar, dairy, meat, alcohol, caffeine and gluten, you want to take at least 7 days to re-introduce these items back in to your diet. (Maybe some of them are gone for good!). DO NOT go out and have a huge steak, 2 martinis, a cup of coffee and a piece of chocolate cake all at the same time!!! I can guarantee that you will not feel so well.

The key to the Refresh Post Week is to take it slow. My advice is to introduce only one item back into your diet each day or two. You will see a Re-Introduction Food Chart at the end of the packet. Use this chart to record your assessment of your body's reaction to the re-introduced food. Do you remember during Week One when I asked you to be more mindful of how you feel after you eat something? Well, during the Refresh Post Week, this is even more important. Be very aware of how your body reacts to the effects of the previously eliminated item. Do you get dizzy from the sugar? Does your heart race after you have the caffeine? Do you feel bloated and sluggish after the red meat? Does the cow's milk or yogurt make your nose stuffy? And does just one glass of wine make you a little tipsy? I suggest you take baby steps and be mindful of not only the physical reactions but also the mental and emotional reactions your body has to the re-introduction of each of the five items.

During the past 3 weeks, a lot of healing took place. I encourage you to go slowly and savor the full benefits of the Refresh. The temptation will be to splurge for all your hard work, but resist. Overloading your system with the foods that you might have been allergic or addicted to can cause severe reactions. Make wise choices and choose what you will be having very carefully. Your body has an innate wisdom, and that wisdom might have been awakened during the Refresh. So pay attention to it as you transition off the Refresh.

Maybe you would like to continue the Refresh a little longer, maybe to reach a desired weight or just because you feel so good! Since this Refresh used a morning smoothie, 'real' food, the daily lemon water, flaxmeal and apple cider vinegar, it actually would not be that difficult to incorporate many of the new practices you have acquired. I do hope that you continue to experiment and get in the kitchen and cook. I wouldn't want you to simply revert directly back to your 'old' ways of eating. You've been down that road before and suffered the consequences of that lifestyle for far too long.

REFRESH POST WEEK GUIDELINES

1. TAKE THE TOXICITY AND INFLAMMATION QUIZ ON PAGE 241 AGAIN.

Record your results in the After column, and compare the results to the Before column. I hope you see the magnitude of your newfound vitality and health! Hopefully, this will inspire you to continue with some of the new eating and lifestyle habits you have obtained during the Refresh.

2. TAKE YOUR VITAL STATISTICS.

Record them again as well. Was there a difference? Did you lose inches? Lose weight? Reduce your BMI?

3. RE-INTRODUCE THE ITEMS YOU HAVE AVOIDED OR ELIMINATED BACK INTO YOUR DAILY DIET.

The next step is to slowly (one item at a time) re-introduce the six items (sugar, caffeine, dairy, meat, alcohol and gluten) back in to your daily diet. (That is, if you choose to. Some of them you might want to take out for good.) Realistically, you should try to introduce one item, let's say sugar, and then take a few days to see how your body reacts. If you are OK, move on to meat, then dairy, etc. By going slowly, and only doing one at a time, you will be able to identify if it is that particular item that might have been giving you problems or creating unfavorable health symptoms for you prior to the Refresh.

4. USE OUR FOOD RE-INTRODUCTION CHART TO TRACK YOUR PROGRESS.

Our Food Rei-Introduction chart will enable you to track any symptoms you experience. Remember, symptoms may occur anywhere from a few minutes to 72 hours after ingestion and can include fatigue, headaches, brain fog, diarrhea, reflux, mood changes, digestive upset, joint pains, fluid retention, changes in sleep patterns, rashes, and much more.

You can download a PDF of the chart from our website at: www.attaintruehealth.com/chart

Make 6 copies of the chart. Label them sugar, caffeine, alcohol, dairy, meat and gluten. For example—on your sugar chart in the food column, make a note if you have a cookie, ice cream, a candy bar, cake, etc., and mark down the time (keeping in mind that a cookie would also be noted on the gluten chart if it contains wheat). Then go across and note how this item made you feel in the following categories:

Pulse

Sit quietly and count your pulse for 60 seconds and write it down. Continue to sit quietly for 20 minutes after introducing the new food, and then count pulse again for 60 seconds and record. Now listen to your body for a moment and see how you are feeling. Any indigestion? Sinus congestion? How is your energy? Please record the significant data onto the chart for your own evaluation.

Indigestion

How does your stomach feel? Any rumbling or gurgling?

Bowel – Did this item make you run to the bathroom or have the opposite effect and constipate you? Some of these categories might take a day or two to see a pattern. That is why it is suggested to only introduce one at a time and give it 1-2 days.

Head/Nasal

Did you get a headache or any congestion after eating this item?

Joints

If your joint aches and pains improved during the Refresh, just note if any item makes the symptoms return.

Kidney/Bladder

Just pay more attention to your bathroom habits and also

be aware of any pain in your lower back/kidney area after introducing an item back.

Energy

This is a big one! Pay close attention to your energy level after re-introducing an item, especially sugary things, bread or any other simple, refined carbohydrate. Do you feel sleepy or that you need a nap an hour later?

(This might seem like a nuisance but it might be the most attention you have paid to the natural workings of your body in a long time!)

5. TRY TO INCORPORATE THE NEW, HEALTHIER FOOD OPTIONS INTO YOUR DAILY ROUTINE.

If at all possible, try to continue the lemon/warm water drink first thing each morning.

Have some fruit for breakfast.

Continue to experiment with your smoothie/protein drink each morning.

Make a habit of adding ground flaxseed to your yogurt, salads or fruit.

The apple cider vinegar will counteract the acidic foods we consume, so keep it up.

Increase your intake of vegetables, especially the dark, green leafy ones!

Experiment with the many new whole grains you haven't tried yet.

Keep filling up your water bottle over the course of the day.

Add any kind of exercise or movement to your daily habits.

Remember to take some very deep breaths during the course of your day.

Try to keep your stress levels down

Form a nighttime ritual to stop eating two hours before bed, exfoliating your skin in a nice hot bath and finding ways to nurture yourself.

6. CONSCIOUSLY GIVE YOURSELF PERMISSION TO MAKE YOUR BODY A PRIORITY.

I do recommend that we Refresh twice a year, so find a friend to join you next time around!

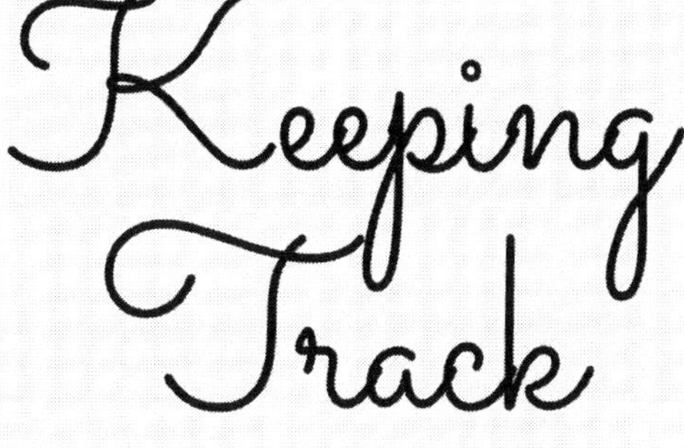

Keeping Track

WEEK ONE
BY THE DAY

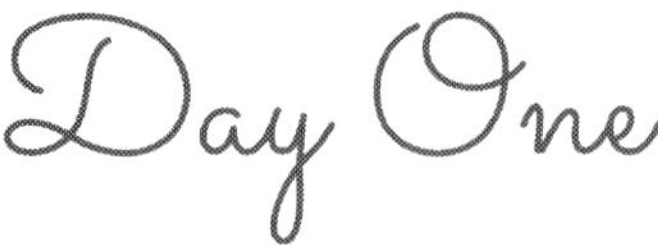

Day One

AND SO WE BEGIN.

It might have been a sacrifice for you over the prep week to 'give up' some foods that you have been dependent upon for years. But stick to it, and soon it won't seem as difficult.

Please take a moment to close your eyes and think about why you are doing this. Whatever your intention is, you are here so that you can make a change in your health and in your life. Pat yourself on the back for taking the first step. Very excited, a little scared and lots of apprehension...all very normal.

This quote by Kareem Abdul Jabar, the famous basketball player, says it all—

"I think that the good and the great are only separated by the willingness to sacrifice."

You've all already proven you are great! Keep up the good work. And at the end of your first day, jot down some thoughts in the space below about how you feel.

DATE:

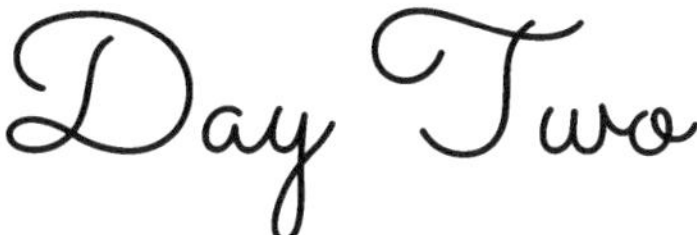

HOW ARE YOU DOING?

There are things that you'll need to do before heading into your day (i.e. lemon water, apple cider vinegar, flax meal, smoothie etc.). Prepare as much as you can the night before and it will soon become part of your natural routine.

Pay close attention to all your feelings and emotions, as well as any physical changes. You might still be feeling the side effects of withdrawal symptoms from the foods you gave up. Don't overdo activities this first week. Rest when possible. Go to bed early. Be mindful of how your body is reacting to all these changes! And make a note of it here.

And remember. It is the little things we do over time that make the biggest changes.

"Lasting change does not happen overnight. Lasting change happens in infinite, similar increments; a day, an hour, a minute, a heartbeat at a time."

~Anonymous

DATE:

Day Three

ARE YOU SHORT ON ENERGY?

While some of us may feel awesome, some of us may be just a wee bit cranky without your usual latte. It's normal to feel a little out of it right now, but I promise, it will pass. If you are hungry, eat more. Real, whole foods, are nutrient dense and lower in calories. Make sure you are getting a wide variety of foods. This quote sums it up!

"Now is no time to think of what you do not have. Think of what you can do with what there is." ~Ernest Hemingway

If you are missing red meat (and the protein and energy it provides), try more legumes, namely lentils, chickpeas, and sweet peas. Lentils are my favorite go-to-dish and so fast and easy to cook. They are an excellent source of protein and iron, which you need plenty of when you aren't eating meat.

Remember to have some type of protein at every meal!

DATE:

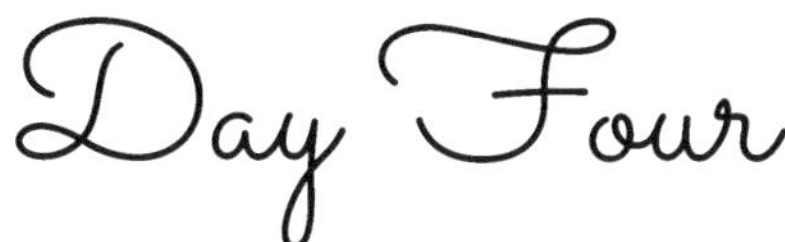

Day Four

TAKE EACH DAY AS IT COMES.

We need to remember to take each day as it comes. One day we might feel unbelievably great and the next, we feel like we will never make another 17 days. But that is what this is all about—progress. One step at a time, we make subtle changes and we see how our body reacts. We will each experience a setback or two, but if we just keep plugging along, we will eventually notice a change.

"I find the great thing in this world is not so much where we stand, as in what direction we are moving. To reach the port of heaven, we must sail sometimes with the wind and sometimes against it - but we must sail, and not drift, nor lie at anchor." ~Oliver Wendell Holmes

To progress we must make an effort. We must forge ahead. We must put ourselves out there and be open to experiences that challenge us. Just look at each day during this Refresh as a challenge. How you react will determine your success.

DATE:

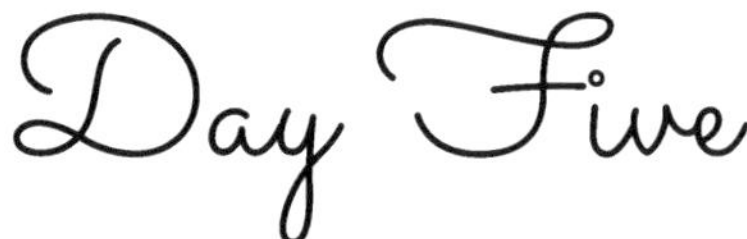

Day Five

CHANGE BRINGS OPPORTUNITY

Do you ever think about change? There is change happening in front of us all the time. There are the changes of the seasons, changes in the landscape as buildings go up and down. Some changes could be called improvements. Recordings went from 8-track to vinyl to cassette to CD to iPods and iPhones. We see the change in people, too. We watched Harry Potter grow up before our very eyes! People change hairstyles, fashion, and addresses.

Change is constant, and it's not like we can or would want to do anything to stop it. There are changes that just happen, and then there are changes that we create for ourselves. I have learned over time that change brings opportunity.

"If nothing ever changed, there would be no butterflies." ~unknown

As we move through the 21 days, reflect on your intention and what you wanted to change about yourself. And then reflect on how you can make that change last.

DATE:

Day Six

A TURNING POINT

Headaches, rashes, low energy, and maybe the overwhelming need for coffee!!! All of this is to be expected. The next day or two will be a turning point for most of you. If you began the process of reducing and eliminating certain foods during the Prep Week, you should be well on your way past the withdrawal stage.

You may be in the thick of the 'toxic reaction' stage!! This too shall pass...but more importantly, if you are having some type of withdrawal, reaction or over-reaction to what's happening to your body, take a moment to contemplate this.

Just think about how addictive that coffee was if your body is screaming for some or how toxic the effects of dairy were if you noticed that your nose has stopped running.

Being mindful of how your body is reacting to not eating the substance you are craving. NOT eating it is the first step in making a change.

If you want a plate of cheese and crackers settle for an orange and some almonds instead. Make choices; see how you react.

If you haven't already, set some goals in the space on the next page of what else you could accomplish during the Refresh besides losing toxins. Weight loss, better clarity, no more aches and pains, more energy.

A goal is different than an intention. Anthony Robbins is a motivational speaker. He always talks about setting goals, looking into the future and making it happen. Here's his quote for the day:

"Setting goals is the first step in turning the invisible into the visible."

If you want it to be visible, you need to write it down so you can 'see' it.

DATE:

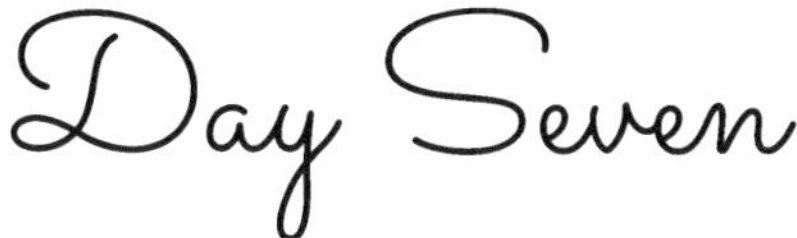

Day Seven

THE END OF WEEK ONE!

Pat yourself on the back, take a bow, and commend yourself for sticking with it.

You may be having difficulty with 'detox' symptoms. Whether it is cold or flu-like symptoms, headaches, aches and pains or lethargy, just know that it will get better as each day passes.

Or you may have already crossed over the hump and are feeling better, with renewed energy and vigor.

Either way, always keep in mind why you did the Refresh in the first place. It will keep you going!

We are one third of the way there so here's my quote for the day: **"When you get into a tight place and everything goes against you, till it seems as though you could not hang on a minute longer, never give up then, for that is just the place and time that the tide will turn."** ~Harriet Beecher Stowe

DATE:

WEEK TWO
BY THE DAY

Day Eight

LIFESTYLE TRANSFORMATION

As we move through Week Two, you may find that you have found your 'groove'. You are feeling good, you are energized, and you realize that some of the small changes you have made have really paid off.

If you are still fighting the 'detox slump' just remember like any marathon, weight loss program, or other long term goal, there is always the hump or plateau we need to 'get over'.

Including the 'Prep Week', you have been working at refreshing your system for two weeks now and it seems like an eternity. It gets harder to stay on track. Your old habits want to creep back in.

However, this is a crucial week—STAY FOCUSED!

The ability to stay disciplined is a trying time. My yoga master describes discipline as the ability to **direct your energy in orderly and organized ways.**

When you set a goal and work toward achieving it, you are exercising your power of self-discipline. That is one of the greatest powers you have! There is no one at your home or at work looking over you. You are doing this Refresh all on your own and it is all up to you whether you stick it out. You have put in effort for two weeks now, and it is worth it.

Self-discipline is the key to success in life! You can master ANYTHING if you are motivated by self-discipline.

You have applied self-discipline in all that you have accomplished thus far in your life.

From something as simple as getting up when the alarm goes off each morning to something not so pleasant as downing your vinegar 'shooter'!

Now I am asking you to incorporate the following lifestyle changes into your daily habits:

- Allow detoxification time before bed
- Practice some movement every day
- Add deep breathing and mindful meditation
- Evaluate personal care products
- Exfoliate dead skin
- Learn ways to de-stress

As important as the food/diet changes you have made over the last two weeks are, these lifestyle habits will 'nourish' you just as much!

"It was character that got us out of bed, commitment that moved us into action, and discipline that enabled us to follow through!" ~Zig Ziglar

DATE:

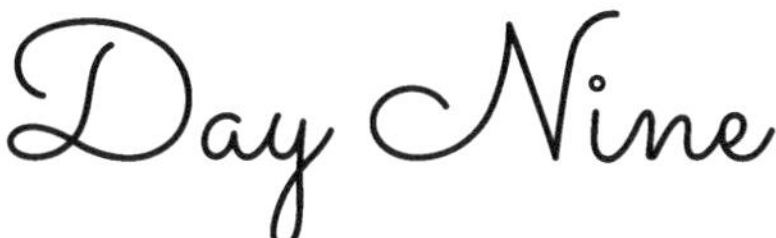

Day Nine

DEEP BREATHING

We will be adding in some lifestyle factors this week that can change everything.

Food is glorious, so keep that up. But now let's focus on a few other things.

Sit up straight, close your eyes and take a deep breath—a really deep breath. In through your nose and then let it out through your mouth with a slow aahhhh. Now just sit for a moment.

Didn't that feel good? You should make a conscious effort to do that more often. Deep breathing allows the body to take in more oxygen and release more carbon dioxide. This leads to many health benefits such as a lowering of blood pressure, slowing of heart rate, and relaxation of the muscles.

It also calms the mind, helps to reduce insomnia, increases your energy, reduces fatigue and eliminates anxiety and stress! Wow...who wouldn't want to take a deep breath every now and then?

How about you make a mindful decision during the Refresh to take three more deep breaths each day; one before breakfast, lunch and dinner? Easy to remember and it might just settle you down enough to enjoy your food more!

I have another breathing technique below that is really good for getting out the toxins and stale air that sits at the bottom of your lungs. It is called Dragon Breath. It's my favorite way of releasing toxic, stale air from my lungs. So try this one tonight.

1) Get down on your hands and knees on the floor.
2) Lift your chin up to open your throat.

3) Close your eyes.

4) Open your mouth very wide, relax your jaw. 5) Inhale a big breath of air and PUSH it out in one big gush like a fire-breathing dragon—you can even make a roaring noise if you want! You'll look really silly but you'll feel really good after your release. Do it three times and then sit back and laugh!

This is the perfect ending to a long day and very detoxifying since it gets the air out from the lowest part of your lungs (which is not circulated as much as we would like since we tend to shallow breathe all day long).

"The most important thing in life is not the triumph but the struggle. The essential thing is not to have conquered but to have fought well." ~Pierre de Courbertin

This week is all about the struggle, the fight to keep on going. If you are dealing with stomach upsets, nausea, or fatigue - listen to your body. Cut back on some things, get more rest, drink lots of water. Make note here of what you ate, how much rest you had and what changed so that you can make corrections for tomorrow.

And keep breathing deeply...

DATE:

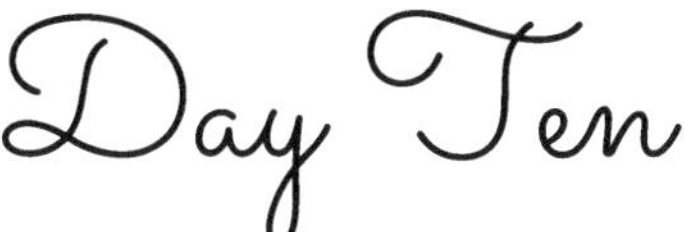

Day Ten

MOVEMENT

In order to properly Refresh your body, you will need to partake in some form of exercise or movement—a good walk will work—not only to stay in shape, but also to encourage circulation and equal distribution of oxygen to your body. Even if you are a little tired, you will find yourself much more likely to be higher in spirits and enthusiasm if you get in some movement. Your skin is a major organ that eliminates toxins from your body and you can double the elimination of toxins by simply sweating and exercising. Remember to wear loose fitting clothes that will allow your skin to sweat and breathe easily.

Exercise and movement are an essential part of your successful Refresh. With a little bit of hard work, you can get your body working just right and free of toxins in no time!

"Winners make goals, losers make excuses." ~Unknown

DATE:

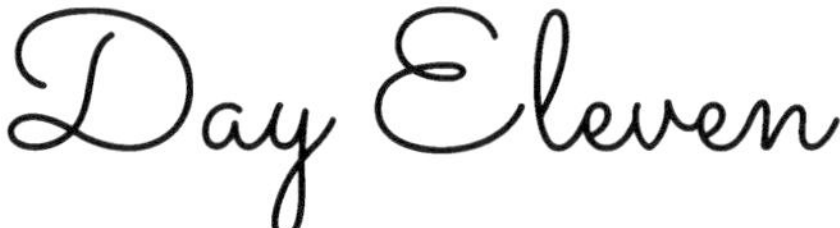

DE-STRESS

Stress is toxic. We are trying to avoid toxins over these 21 days! So be proactive. Identify your 'triggers' and then work out what to do about them. If you know there are certain things, people or circumstances that stress you out, maybe during the Refresh, you can focus on the results you want instead of what is stressing you out. Picture yourself relaxing, meeting your deadline, or getting a good night's sleep—instead of envisioning everything going wrong. Use meditation or a candle flame to focus your thoughts. Even if your mind is active and it takes a while to calm down, just the process of sitting down and managing to slow your breath down is a great form of de-stressing.

"Every area of trouble gives out a ray of hope, and the one unchangeable certainty is that nothing is certain or unchangeable." ~John F. Kennedy

DATE:

Day Twelve

EXFOLIATION

You might be experiencing hives, rashes, bumps and skin break-outs. As I mentioned, our skin is our biggest elimination organ. It releases a pound of waste per day and is the first organ to show symptoms of imbalance or toxicity.

If toxins are unable to escape through the skin, they will either be stored once again in your fat cells or they will be re-circulated back into the blood stream, overworking the kidneys, liver and other detox organs. Thus, a seemingly simple and easy therapy like dry skin brushing can have a huge overall impact on your whole body's health.

Take a long, hot bath which allows for the pores to open and release extra toxins. While bathing, wet brushing is not only detoxifying but it is a great stress reliever too. This week is all about pampering yourself!

"The secret of health for both mind and body is not to mourn the past, nor to worry about the future, but to live the present moment wisely and earnestly." ~Buddha

DATE:

Day Thirteen

PERSONAL CARE

Schedule self-care into your day—put it on your calendar. You will find that doing something specifically for yourself sends a message to you and your body of its intrinsic value. You will find yourself making decisions throughout your day that support your true needs rather than what others expect of you. Especially during the Refresh, it is important to take care of your body. It has been taking care of you for a long time. Go get a massage, a manicure, take a walk in the park just to smell the fresh air. Put your feet up and call a friend whom you haven't talked to in a while and tell her what you are doing and how the Refresh is going.

Read a book with a sparkling glass of seltzer with some pomegranate juice added in. Watch a sitcom on TV and have some deep belly laughs. Play with the dog or your children and just take a moment to be grateful for all that you have. You can even write a gratitude in the space below.

Gratitude is a quality similar to electricity: it must be produced and discharged and used up in order to exist at all.
~William Faulkner

DATE:

Day Fourteen

END OF WEEK 2

You have come a long way. You will probably be amazed by your new passion for your health.

Passion is a primal human trait. Whether it is passion for a person, place or an activity like cooking, It is the passion that carries us forward to new and greater heights of life experiences. And it is through these experiences that we learn more about ourselves. So it is with this Refresh. Now...on to the final week!

"Without passion man is a mere latent force and possibility, like flint which awaits the shock of iron before it can give forth its spark." -Henri Amiel

DATE:

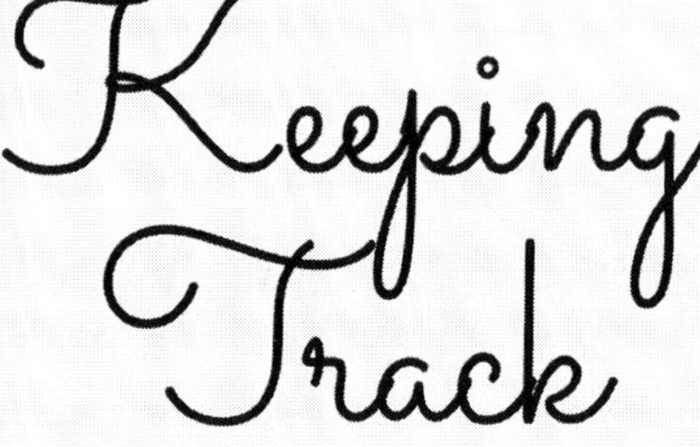

WEEK THREE
BY THE DAY

Day Fifteen

RAW FOOD

Food is fuel for the body, right? Aside from eating food because it tastes delicious and makes you feel good, the primary reason we consume food is to provide us with energy. Raw food like fresh vegetables, fruit, nuts, seeds, seaweeds, sprouts and superfoods contains the nutrients your body seeks daily for nourishment, along with the enzymes your body needs to break down the food and assimilate it.

This week I invite you to incorporate uncooked food at every meal, thus ensuring that you have the elements your body needs to properly digest the food (enzymes) and give you life force energy, nourishing you on a deep cellular level. Not only will your energy soar, but your body will naturally begin to function at an optimal level, thus you will feel like you can do anything!

By now, during this third week, your body should be ready to accept more raw foods. Your system has been 'cleaned' out a bit and it is now prepared for more enzymatic activity. If you are presently just eating more salads or a bowl of fruit in the morning—that's great! But there are other ways to add in more RAW: Go to the local farmer's market or health food store and purchase the veggies and fruits that are in season. This way, you'll see an amazing array of colors change on your plate as the seasons turn. Experiment with some you have never had before. Use your blender (or a juicer if you have one) to make exotic drinks and I don't mean Margaritas! Your morning smoothies are satisfying and delicious; why not add a veggie/fruit spritzer in the afternoon when you come home from work? Blend your favorites, think outside the box (using cucumber, celery, cherries, mango etc.) and mix them with sparkling water when they are done blending. Then take a deep breath and sit down to enjoy it!

Add more vegetables, nuts and sprouts into your wraps, salads and cold pasta or grains. More than you ever thought you would! I enjoy crunch so raw is my go-to instead of chips! Experiment with the recipes I gave you or just google 'raw food recipes' and you will be AMAZED at the thousands of ideas! Keep up the momentum - you are doing exactly what you are supposed to be. This is our FINAL week and you will be surprised at all that will continue to happen for you if you just stay present. Don't look back, we are moving forward!

"Hope is like the sun, which, as we journey toward it, casts the shadow of our burden behind us." ~Samuel Smiles~

DATE:

Day Sixteen

FERMENTED FOOD

Adding more fermented foods into your diet is extremely beneficial. Most fermented foods are now considered to be "probiotics," because they promote the growth of friendly intestinal bacteria. They also increase your overall nutritional benefits by allowing you to absorb your nutrients more readily. They aid in building your immune function and lowering your cholesterol.

For some of you, the process of preparing your own and then waiting for them could be annoying. However, the benefits outweigh the aggravation. It is getting easier to find real fermented and cultured foods in the grocery store now.

If you don't think you have the time to make the fermented recipes later in this book, at least try to up your consumption of some of the most common fermented foods found in the grocery store such as soy sauce, miso, tempeh or sheep, goat or coconut yogurt this week to get some of the benefits. And also remember that you are getting your daily dose of probiotics in your morning Shaklee Life Shakes. One billion CFU's of probiotic along with the prebiotics to feed them!

Today's thought: **"People often say that motivation doesn't last. Well, neither does bathing—that's why we recommend it daily."** ~ Zig Ziglar

DATE:

Day Seventeen

KEEP GOING...

We are nearing the end! You should have found the changes in your daily eating habits working well for you, especially with the lemon water, flaxseeds and apple cider vinegar. Those things alone will make an impact on your health. You have worked hard over the last few weeks. It has taken perseverance, diligence and sheer willpower at times. This might be a nice time to decide what your 'reward' will be once you have successfully completed the 21 days. Maybe a massage or a new hairstyle. I don't reward myself with food. Have you ever noticed that sometimes you eat something because you've craved it for so long and then it just doesn't do the trick of satisfying that craving? That is just one of the many rewards of this Refresh!

"The reward of a thing well done is to have done it." ~Ralph Waldo Emerson

DATE:

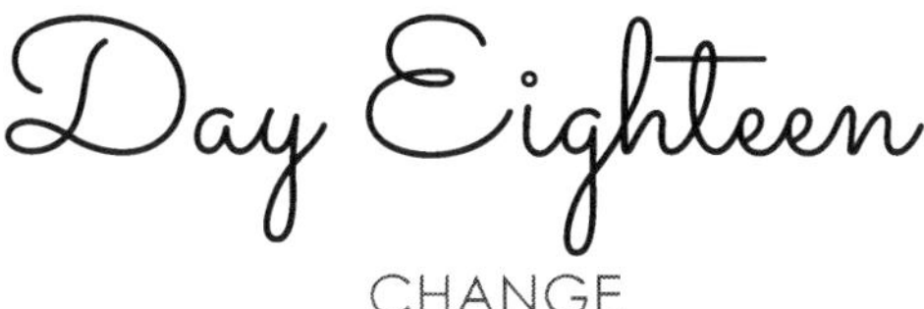

Day Eighteen

CHANGE

Has anything about your life, your body, your health or your attitude changed over the last few weeks? Do you think you can make lasting change? We tend to assume that circumstances change easily and often, but that people change rarely, slowly, and with great difficulty. But these assumptions are wrong. The truth is that people can change easily and instantly. The real problem is that they also change back just as easily! Meanwhile, the circumstances of our lives change slowly in comparison. If you're fifty pounds overweight, and you just changed your eating habits, it's going to take a while before the change in your habits shows up on your body. And if you decide that your new habits aren't helping, you just might change them back! At the beginning of this Refresh I asked you to be mindful. Now I am asking you to jot down all the things you noticed. It can be as simple as "I am sleeping better" or as remarkable as " I didn't think I could go without coffee but now I don't even want it anymore!"

"Everyone thinks of changing the world, but no one thinks of changing himself." ~Leo Nikolaevich Tolstoy

DATE:

Day Nineteen

YOU NOW HAVE A FOUNDATION TO BUILD FROM...

If you have truly gone 18 days without sugar, you are to be commended! Living without processed sugar can be incredibly rewarding. It's almost a surefire way to have more energy, boost your immune system and improve your moods. The good news is that once you wean yourself off sugar, you can learn to eat a little here and there without getting sucked into the sugar addiction vortex all over again. For now, we're doing without so your body learns what it's like to be sugar-free. This is important work, so stick with it. Some of the recipes in this book are desserts—in an attempt to show you that we don't need the refined, sugary sweets from the grocery store. We are using some of the natural sugars from Mother Nature such as honey, maple syrup, dates and Stevia. If refined sugar was your biggest obstacle and you succeeded in eliminating it, just think what else you are capable of!

"There are four pillars on which you can build the platform to reach the zenith of success: Dedication, Devotion, Discipline and Determination." ~Lakkoju Goutam

DATE:

Day Twenty

MOMENTUM

Momentum is a commonly used term in sports. A team that has momentum is on the move and is going to take some effort to stop. For you on this Refresh, momentum means progress: amazing sleep, loss of sugar cravings, waking up feeling great, cooking more and feeling energized.

Do you want to keep the momentum going?

If you are at that point where you have made significant improvements in your health but just don't know if you can keep it going, then there is the option of working with me privately to keep the momentum going.

My program is designed to educate, inform, support and guide you so that after an additional 90 days, you have the tools you need to carry this out for the rest of your life. And first and foremost, by participating in my programs - there is NO deprivation. All the foods you reduced or eliminated in the Refresh are back in, if you choose them to be. For those of you that might need some additional support and guidance regarding your eating habits, your fear of going back to your old ways, losing more weight, or keeping up with healthy lifestyle choices after this Refresh is over, then my Programs are for you. You have made the initial commitment during the past 21 days, which means you are in the perfect place to make the mindset shift which is what is required now to continue to move forward.

For those of you that need 'specialized' assistance and would like to keep your journey going, please check out my varied programs by going to: www.attaintruehealth.com

"Creating a beautiful life is your highest calling. Celebrate this new awareness. It is in the details of life that beauty is

revealed, sustained and nurtured." ~Anonymous

DATE:

Day Twenty-One

YOU DID IT!

You are either saying "Thank goodness, I never thought this day would come!" or you are embracing the fact that you never imagined you could do it and here it is…and now you feel a tremendous sense of accomplishment. Either way, my hope is that you learned something over the past few weeks. You began this journey for a reason. Sit back and analyze the outcome. Did you accomplish what you set out to do? Did you learn something about yourself that you never expected? And most importantly, did your body thank you?

Whatever it is you take with you, give yourself a round of applause for the journey. You may have had ups and downs throughout the Refresh. Temptation abounds and whether you gave in to temptation or not—it's all about what you learned from the experience. Our lives are about balance. We all know what we should be eating, how much and when.

But I believe in the 80-20 rule. 80% of the time I stick with what I know is best for my body, cooking more at home, eating organic, monitoring my sugar intake etc. But I am a firm believer that deprivation doesn't work in the long run; it makes you want that 'something' even more. So 20% of the time, I give in—going out to restaurants and splurging, eating a little dark chocolate and indulging in macaroni and cheese (my weakness!); good quality with 4 cheeses and not made from a box, of course.

It is important that our lives and our health are balanced. 100 calories of cake is not the same as 100 calories of organic blueberries. If you continue to eat quality, highly nutritious calories (by choosing more organic food, meat that hasn't been injected with hormones, etc.), the easier it will be for your body to balance itself out. Just remember the 80-20 rule and try not to stress yourself out.

The Refresh Post Week is just as important as the past 21 days. Take today as your last full day on the Refresh so look for ways to slowly re-introduce foods back into your daily eating habits using the guidelines provided.

"The needle of our conscience is as good a compass as any." ~Ruth Wolff

DATE:

Frequently Asked Questions

What can I expect during the Refresh?

This is a time to concentrate on YOU. Most of you will see an immediate improvement in your overall health, less aches and pains, effortless weight loss, clearer skin, less wrinkles, an abundance of energy, lack of need for sleep, and an overall youthful appearance.

You will find any ailments will begin to improve as your body begins to take on the life force energy of real foods. You will be eating a lot less foods that are allergenic, acidic or addictive.

What do I have to give up?

It is recommended to remove gluten, dairy, refined sugars, red meat, pork, alcohol, and caffeine from your diet.

What will I gain?

A better understanding of food and cooking, as well as how certain foods make your body feel better or worse. How to make the best choices for yourself. And you will also gain a more mindful approach to everyday life.

Will I lose weight?

Many people often lose weight on the Refresh as the toxins begin to leave the body and you start putting the proper 'fuel' inside on a daily basis. It allows your body to come back in to balance.

Will I have enough to eat?

Absolutely. This Refresh includes over 125 original food and smoothie recipes, daily meal planning guides and grocery lists. Refreshers in the past have often remarked that they've felt full and satisfied every day.

Why is this Refresh different?

By using the standard methods of an elimination diet AND adding in the Shaklee Life Shake and some enhancing supplements AND becoming more mindful of your body in general, this is a winning combination. When we allow the body to be free of the additional toxic overload from the foods on the 'avoid' list, it starts to use its own natural detoxification systems, bringing the body back into balance. And then the Life Shake provides added support for our gut health with one billion CFU's (Colony Forming Units) of probiotics to replenish our gut flora and the prebiotic to feed those probiotics. Plus, the recommended supplements will complete the overall detoxification and free up the body to be fully Refreshed!

How will I ever give up coffee and wine?

I have heard this remark so many times. Not surprisingly, people are very hesitant to give up the things they love. I've found people often don't give a second thought to cutting out gluten, dairy, or meat. But coffee and wine (alcohol) are another story because both of these are addictive and a huge part of our social culture.

The reason we stop coffee besides being addictive is that it is highly acidic and we are trying to alkalize ourselves during the Refresh. I understand that coffee is a ritual for many and you feel very attached to it. This is where mindfulness comes in. Do you drink it because your parents did and you grew up with it? Because you like the taste? Because you can't start your day without that burst of energy? All of these reasons are valid but please re-access your 'why'.

I have had many, many people tell me that they would not participate in the Refresh because there was no way they would give up their coffee. But I convinced them and they tried. The Refresh means you might have to break your daily habits. But amazing things happen. Those participants who gave up coffee found their own energy levels and had better mental clarity. Once weaned, they realized if they were tired it was because their body was really tired, not because they did not have their caffeine that day. I encourage you to go for it.

And as far as alcohol is concerned, it's liquid sugar. Grab a pretty glass and add your seltzer with lemon and get on with it for 21 days. Your body will thank you and your face will show the most improvement. No alcohol for 21 days and those bags under your eyes go away. And you will lose some weight —guaranteed.

After the Refresh, if you resume drinking coffee or wine, you might find that you don't crave it as much or drink nearly as much as before. Bonus!

Will the results last?

The Refresh will teach you not only a new way to eat but also a new lifestyle. Often, participants will adapt the Refresh guidelines to fit their daily lifestyle and continue to change their eating habits because they just feel that great!

I eat pretty healthy. How do I begin the Refresh?

The first step is to clean house. It's best to start with the 'foods to avoid' section on pages 20 , but for now take a look inside your refrigerator and pantry and remove all processed or manufactured foods. And if you already eat healthy, it is all about the small changes and the mindfulness with your choices that is going to make the biggest changes for you during the Refresh.

What are the essentials I must have in my home in order to get started?

It's hard to say how much of a transition this will be for you, since I don't know what your pantry looks like. But the minimum kitchen tools you will need are a decent blender, food processor, a sharp knife and cutting board. That's a good start!

As you become more committed to your lifestyle, your

needs may change.

As for food items, simple is best. Since you are about to clean out your pantry of old processed foods that will no longer be necessary, please check out the Staples Checklist on page 32 and review your needs based on what you have in your pantry. Most importantly, though, purchase mostly real, plant food, some chicken and fish and the required protein powder and supplements.

I'm used to eggs, toast, or cereal for breakfast. What should I eat now?

Smoothies are a requirement on the Refresh. Starting your day off with an energy boost and not something that will weigh you down, I always think smoothies! Everybody loves smoothies, but we seem to have a mental block against considering them as a meal since many people categorize them in the "drink" department. The Shaklee Life Energizing Shake is a full, satisfying meal. Blending in your daily greens, along with fruit, nuts, seeds and spices will help the vitamins and minerals absorb quickly and make it an enjoyable breakfast to wake up to. (See Recipes for great smoothie ideas.)

What about supplements?

It is a known fact that foods today do not provide enough nutritional value. Our soils are depleted, we are fractionating and genetically modifying our foods and there are just too many artificial ingredients, preservatives etc. in the foods we eat. I like to think of the supplements I take as Superfoods. Research has shown that we cannot get our required nutrients in just the foods we eat. Mark Hyman, MD said it best -

"(You don't need a supplement) ONLY if you eat wild, fresh, whole, organic, local, non-genetically modified food grown in virgin mineral and nutrient soils, and not transported across vast distances and stored for months before eaten...work and live outside, breathe only fresh unpolluted air, drink only pure, clean water, sleep nine hours a night, move your body every day, and are free from chronic stressors and exposures to environmental toxins."

So if you fit all those requirements, then no supplementation is necessary!

I love to eat out. Can I dine out during the Refresh?

Dining out is a wonderful way to meet friends, not have to cook, and experience cuisine you might not make at home. I highly encourage you to eat out during the Refresh. It can be a social experience or a culinary delight but once again, making mindful choices is the key. Restaurants are very accommodating today and usually don't mind questions about whether a dish has gluten or dairy etc.

I get low blood sugar. Are you sure I'll be okay on the Refresh?

As your body detoxifies, your blood sugar will begin to level out and you will no longer experience blood sugar lows. One of the most noticeable changes when you introduce more real food into your diet is the amount of food you will need. You will discover that you automatically adjust to a different pace or interval of eating. You may have been used to eating three large meals, but will find you adjust to consuming less food more often throughout the day. On the Refresh, you eat more real foods and less processed foods or what I call 'empty calories'. Your body will feel full and nourished more quickly as you are receiving more nutrients per mouthful. This shift is not only easier on your digestive tract, but will ultimately speed up your metabolism as your body is working more efficiently. Listen to your body—it will let you know what it needs.

What is a toxin and how did I get them in my body?

Any kind of substance that is harmful to your body may be considered a toxin. There are a variety of toxins from the environment that we cannot help but be affected by. These include pollution, car exhaust, disease-causing bacteria and non-naturally occurring chemical substances. And then there are also toxins in our foods such as preservatives, additives, artificial sweeteners, waxes, dyes, artificial flavors and colorings. So as you can see, it is not difficult to create a toxic environment in our body. And lastly, there are the toxins you get through your skin from your moisturizer, shampoo, conditioners, make-up, perfumes etc.

Who is encouraged to do a Refresh?

Our body is constantly refreshing, cleansing and detoxifying itself every day, which in turn allows us to stay well balanced, often referred to as homeostasis. When we are exposed to a multitude of toxins, we store them in our fat cells, tissues, and other organs. Even antibiotics from your youth or the build up fast food chemicals can stay in your body for long periods of time. Therefore, the body is not able to maintain balance. In these instances, doing a Refresh that allows us to detoxify will certainly help the body to Refresh and then balance itself, eliminating the cause of disease before illness manifests. The majority of us can usually benefit from the rest to the body that this Refresh will provide. It provides your body with a 'service and a tune-up' just as you would give your car a service when it is not running smoothly. So everyone is encouraged to do a Refresh one to two times a year to keep the toxic load at a minimum.

What precautions and safeguards should I take?

You should not undertake this Refresh without having first obtained professional advice:

* If you are pregnant and/or breast-feeding a baby.

* Before or shortly after any major surgery when the body is weak

* If you suffer from any long-term physical or mental

illness, or if you are undertaking treatment for cancer

* If you are under 18 years or over 65 years of age

* You should consult with your doctor about any kind of medications that were prescribed by your doctor for you. We are only eating real foods and using supplements that are pure, so there should not be any conflicts but please check.

* If you take medication as a diabetic, it is important to continue to monitor your blood sugar frequently while on the Refresh.

What happen if I eat something I am not supposed to?

Don't worry about it! Just don't make a habit of it. The purpose of the Refresh is to change your eating habits. It might be difficult at first, but the benefits outweigh the detriments.

If you have a special event, wedding or party to go to, just be aware of what you are eating. Make different choices than you would have in the past. Being mindful about what we consume is the first step in the right direction.

And if you slip up with a bowl of ice cream one night, get back on track the following morning.

Keeping in touch with your fellow Refreshers on the online forum will be a great asset. Then you will see that you are not the only one who might have had that bowl of ice cream.

Just do the best you can!

Bear in Mind...

A few things to bear in mind.

IF YOU FEEL TIRED, DIZZY OR WEAK. Eat more. The Attain True Health Refresh has nothing to do with counting calories or restricting portions. Eat plenty of beans, nuts and healthy fats in your diet. Feel free to include more chicken and fish. Also, be sure you are getting enough sleep. This is the perfect time to get more rest.

IF YOU HAVE GAS OR BLOATING. Many of you will have no trouble at all since you are eating a lot more fruits and vegetables. However, gas happens...especially if you are not used to eating real food; your body is more used to digesting pizza than kale. Try to pay attention and avoid the foods that cause the worst symptoms. Just remember, the food on this Refresh is the kind of food your body was meant to digest; it just might take yours a little longer to realize that. Also, the kombu suggestion in the basic bean recipe assists with gas.
And, maybe you need to order some EZ-Gest (Item #20633 from my website at www.alysonchugerman.myshaklee.com or through your own Shaklee distributor's website). This will introduce more digestive enzymes into your system and allow you to better absorb and process your food.

IF YOU JUST GENERALLY DON'T FEEL WELL. If it is serious, please see a doctor. Otherwise, please email my team at support@attaintruehealth.com with your symptoms and we will try to troubleshoot your problem.

Sample Menus

Menus for cooler weather

Most of the recipe suggestions on the next few pages can be found in the Recipe Section. When you prepare menu ideas, make sure to make enough for leftovers!

Day 1:

Breakfast	Protein Smoothie, Flax Breakfast Pudding, fresh fruit
Lunch	Warm Spinach Salad with Tuna
Dinner	Stuffed Autumn Squash Sautéed Escarole with Sundried Tomatoes
Dessert	Apple Pumpkin Spice Cake

Day 2:

Breakfast	Protein Smoothie, Pineapple Coconut Yogurt, multi- grain toast, 'healthy' jam
Lunch	Tabouli Salad
Dinner	Fish Tacos with Melon Salsa, Bean Salad
Dessert	Chia Cream

Day 3:

Breakfast	Protein Smoothie, Black Bean Breakfast Burrito, fresh fruit
Lunch	Warm Lentil, Grape, Mint and Feta Salad
Dinner	Honey Garlic Chicken, Chickpea and Raisin Salad, Brown Rice

Day 4:

Breakfast	Protein Smoothie, Brown Rice Porridge, fresh fruit
Lunch	Beet, Carrot, Pear Salad with Rice Cakes
Dinner	Chunky Vegetable Lentil Soup, Creamy Sesame Greens, whole grain bread
Dessert	Apple Bread Pudding

Day 5:

Breakfast	Protein Smoothie, Morning Glory Muffin, fresh fruit
Lunch	Red Cabbage and Grapefruit Salad OR

Basic Rice Bowl
Dinner Bean and Vegetable Stew with Dumplings, Creamed Kale

Day 6:
Breakfast Protein Smoothie, Homemade Granola with healthy milk, fresh fruit
Lunch Roasted vegetables in a wrap/on a salad i.e. beets, brussel sprouts, carrots etc.
Dinner Portobello Curry with Green Rice, salad

Day 7:
Breakfast Protein Smoothie, Alyson's Mediterranean Breakfast
Lunch Green Bean Slaw (make ahead) and Broccoli Soup
Dinner Italian Tofu Frittata, Baked Parmesan Tomatoes
Dessert Chocolate Cherry Cookies

Note: Breakfast selections for Week Two and Three remain the same as Week One

Day 8:
Lunch Mediterranean Lentil Salad, rice cakes
Dinner Quick Broiled Chicken, Sweet Potato Salad with Orange Maple Dressing, sautéed dark leafy greens (Swiss Chard)

Day 9:
Lunch Hearty Greens Soup
Dinner Lemon Tofu, Quinoa with Vinaigrette, Fennel with Raisins and Pine Nuts
Dessert Fried Peanut Butter Bananas

Day 10:
Lunch Quinoa Salad with Black Beans (use leftover quinoa)
Dinner Poached Eggs on Collard Greens/ Shitakes, Arugula Salad with Walnut Croutons

This Refresh was fabulous. I had never done a Refresh before because the first thing that used to come to my mind was that I'd have to drink a bunch of odd-tasting liquids and stay off foods that I love. While I did have to eliminate certain things, Alyson takes a very balanced approach. She provided the tools needed to set me up for success—her recipes are delicious and easy to prepare and they incorporate many of the foods that I already enjoy. She offers motivation and inspiration on a daily basis. Before the Refresh, I ate chocolate every single day and laughed at the possibility of my chocolate cravings disappearing; I didn't think it was possible. I eased in by creating tasty chocolate treats that were sweet, but without refined sugar and by week 2, I was able to go several days without any sugar at all–it was amazing! My energy levels also increased. I'd recommend this Refresh to anyone who is looking to reduce sugar intake and to get on the path to developing healthier eating habits.

–*Gayle B.*

Day 11:

Lunch	Salad or any leftovers
Dinner	Asian Meatball Soup with Kale, Napa Cabbage Salad

Day 12:

Lunch	Golden Butternut Squash Soup, whole grain bread, apple slices
Dinner	Stir-Fried Shrimp with Asparagus, salad
Dessert	Cranberry and Fresh Pear Cobbler

Day 13:

Lunch	Leftover soups or salads
Dinner	Spaghetti Squash Primavera

Day 14:

Lunch	Veggie Tacos with Corn Tortillas
Dinner	Zesty Mexican Soup, salad with fresh corn
Dessert	Orange Coconut Treat

Day 15:

Lunch	Spinach Beet Berry Salad
Dinner	Black Bean Burgers with Peach Salsa, Millet Pilaf, Bok Choy, Sesame Orange Dressing

Day 16:

Lunch	Fruited Celery Salad
Dinner	Miso Salmon, 7 Minute Butternut Squash, grain of your choice

Day 17:

Lunch	Tomato Basil Soup, Kale Salad
Dinner	Raw Pad Thai, Pickled Cucumbers

Day 18:

Lunch	Asian Cabbage and Peanut Salad
Dinner	Swiss Chards Wrap, Basic Miso Soup

Day 19:
Lunch Miso Avocado Sandwich
Dinner Primavera Verde, salad

Day 20:
Lunch Pineapple and Cucumber Gazpacho
Dinner Brown Rice and Goat Cheese Cakes, Root Vegetable Fries with Gremolata, green vegetable of your choice

Day 21:
Lunch Garlic Shrimp Salad
Dinner Green Chicken Chili with Kale, brown rice

Menus for warmer weather

Day 1:
Breakfast Protein Smoothie, Simple Buckwheat Porridge
Lunch Dynasty Salad
Dinner Asian Stuffed Cabbage Rolls, Spinach and Persimmon Salad

Day 2:
Breakfast Protein Smoothie, Superfood Cereal
Lunch Herbed Watermelon Salad
Dinner Grilled Black Bean Burger, Coconut Lime Rice Salad
Dessert Fried Peanut Butter Bananas

Day 3:
Breakfast Protein Smoothie, Apple Raisin Quinoa
Lunch Asparagus Ribbon Salad
Dinner Green Curry and Coconut Soba Noodles, Salad

Day 4:
Breakfast Protein Smoothie, gluten free cereal of your choice with fruit
Lunch Quinoa Bowl, rice crackers
Dinner Shrimp Tacos with Citrus Slaw, Calabacitas
Dessert Cantaloupe Mint Paletas (Ice Pops)

Day 5:
Breakfast Protein Smoothie, Japanese Style Rice Porridge
Lunch Grapefruit Arugula Salad
Dinner Avocado Pesto Pasta, green beans

Day 6:
Breakfast Protein Smoothie, fresh fruit with non-dairy yogurt
Lunch Basic Rice Bowl – choose your veggies!
Dinner Fresh Pea Soup, salad, gluten free bread with coconut oil, salad

Day 7:

Breakfast	Protein Smoothie, scrambled eggs, gluten free toast
Lunch	Mediterranean Quinoa Salad
Dinner	Pan-Seared Cod with Roasted Asparagus
Dessert	The Best Part of Pie

Note: Breakfast selections for Week Two and Three remain the same as Week One

Day 8:

Lunch	Creamy Honey Dijon Salad
Dinner	Orange Chicken Soba Noodles, Roasted Radishes and Leeks
Dessert	Chocolate Chia Pudding

Day 9:

Lunch	Creamy Radish Soup, Snap Pea and Quinoa Salad
Dinner	Fish of your choice, side salad, Garlic Gingered Broccoli

Day 10:

Lunch	Hearty Greens Soup
Dinner	Vegan Macaroni and Cheese, Salad

Day 11:

Lunch	Black Bean Lettuce Wraps
Dinner	Asparagus, Pea and Leek Stir-Fry, Cucumber Salad

Day 12:

Lunch	Mediterranean Lentil Salad
Dinner	Sweet Potatoes with Citrus Ginger Vinaigrette

Day 13:
Lunch Artichoke Leek Soup, salad of your choice
Dinner Marinated Portobello Mushrooms Stuffed with Spinach
Dessert Orange and Coconut Treat

Day 14:
Lunch Leftover soup or salad of your choice
Dinner Asian Tuna Steaks, Napa Cabbage Salad, grain of your choice

Day 15:
Lunch Asian Cabbage Peanut Salad
Dinner Miso Soup with Garlic Shrimp Salad

Day 16:
Lunch Tomato Basil Soup
Dinner Falafel Burgers with Tzatziki and side of Apple Beet Relish

Day 17:
Lunch Wilted Kale Salad with Creamy Chipotle Dressing.
Dinner Mushroom, Tomato and Basil Frittata with Kiwi Salad

Day 18:
Lunch Lemony Cabbage Avocado Slaw
Dinner Vegetable Tofu Stir Fry over brown rice

Day 19:
Lunch Miso Avocado Open-Faced Sandwich
Dinner Lemon Ginger Chicken, smashed potatoes and green beans

I was feeling unhappy with my weight and knew I needed to lose. I was overweight and feeling uncomfortable in my clothes. I was not a fast-food- eater or junk-food- junkie, but did have some issues with portion control and ice cream! I was taking Nexium for years and wanted to eliminate it. I was weaning myself off of it when my friend introduced me to the Refresh. Just give it a try! I did and I am glad I did! Alyson's guidelines, recipes, and inspirational messages helped to make me successful! There was more than enough food to eat and NO counting calories! It felt good to know that I was eating food that my body liked, not just what I liked. I lost weight, was never hungry, eliminated Nexium completely and feel better in general. The Refresh jump-started a lifestyle I knew I needed to achieve and gave me the inspiration and will-power to continue long after the three weeks were over.

–Karen H.

Day 20:

Lunch Strawberry and Fava Bean Salad

Dinner Halibut with Pomegranate Glaze, Millet Pilaf, grilled zucchini

Day 21:

Lunch Romaine Lettuce Wraps

Dinner Lentil Shepherd's Pie, salad

Shopping List

SUGGESTED SHOPPING LIST

Again, you will have to go to the store more than once this week. If I gave you the complete grocery list for each recipe, it would be too overwhelming and too much to buy in one trip. So I have made some reminders of things to check off to make sure you don't run out of them. And then you will need to pick and choose which recipes you will cook for about 3-4 days, make your master list and then do it all over again mid- week with the rest of the recipes.

_____ Check your lemon supply

_____ Check your grain supply; try buckwheat or amaranth from the bulk bin.

_____Check your dark green leafy vegetable supply and aim to add more kale, Swiss chard, arugula, broccoli, Bok Choy, cucumber, celery, avocado, asparagus, spinach

_____Check nut supply; recipes call for almonds, walnuts

Ginger
Garlic
Peppers
Tomatoes
Scallions
Some citrus - grapefruits, oranges, limes
Check out new fruits—papaya, mango, pineapple
Use frozen fruits in your smoothies
Dried fruits such as raisins, prunes, apricots, cranberries
Fresh herbs such as cilantro, parsley, thyme, basil
Scallions
Roasted red peppers

SHOULD I GO ORGANIC? THE CLEAN FIFTEEN AND THE DIRTY DOZEN

The Dirty Dozen.

This is the list of produce you should buy only in organically grown form. According to EWG, (Environmental Working Group) common growing practices make the crops listed below the most likely to contain higher pesticide residues:

1. Strawberries
2. Apples
3. Nectarines
4. Peaches
5. Celery
6. Grapes
7. Cherries
8. Spinach
9. Tomatoes
10. Sweet Bell Peppers
11. Cherry Tomatoes
12. Cucumbers

Also on the list are kale/collard greens and hot peppers which may contain organophosphate insecticides. The EWG characterizes them as "highly toxic" and of special concern.

The Clean Fifteen.

When grown conventionally, the produce on this list poses the least risk of exposure to pesticides. While I always recommend eating organic fruits and vegetables, they may be too expensive for those on tight budgets or simply not available. I encourage everyone to enjoy these fruits and vegetables in organic or conventionally grown form:

1. Avocados
2. Sweet corn
3. Pineapples
4. Cabbage
5. Sweet peas (frozen)
6. Onions
7. Asparagus
8. Mangos
9. Papayas
10. Kiwi
11. Eggplant
12. Honeydew Melon
13. Grapefruit
14. Cantaloupe
15. Cauliflower

Information from the Environmental Working Group
Ewg.org

Recipes

From basic to innovative, these recipes fit all the standards of the Attain True Health Refresh. You can use them anytime, even long after the 21 days are over. Get cookin' and see how delicious and easy real, clean, wholesome food can be!

THE BASICS

Basic Brown Rice

Brown rice has a coating on it called phytic acid. It is best to rinse the rice before use for ease of digestion. Another option is to soak the rice overnight in water with a splash of apple cider vinegar. Before cooking, drain and rinse.

1 cup brown rice
2 cups water

1. Combine the rice and water in a pot.
2. Bring it to a boil, then simmer uncovered until all water is absorbed. *Serves 4*

Basic Quinoa

1 cup quinoa
2 cups water

1. Rinse quinoa to remove a coating of saponin.
2. Combine quinoa and water.
3. Bring to a boil and simmer uncovered until all water is absorbed. *Serves 4*

Basic Millet

1 cup millet
3 cups water

1. Combine millet with water in a pot.
2. Bring to a boil and simmer uncovered until water is absorbed.
   (*Optional*–you can soak millet overnight in water with a splash of apple cider vinegar. Before cooking, drain and rinse). *Serves 4*

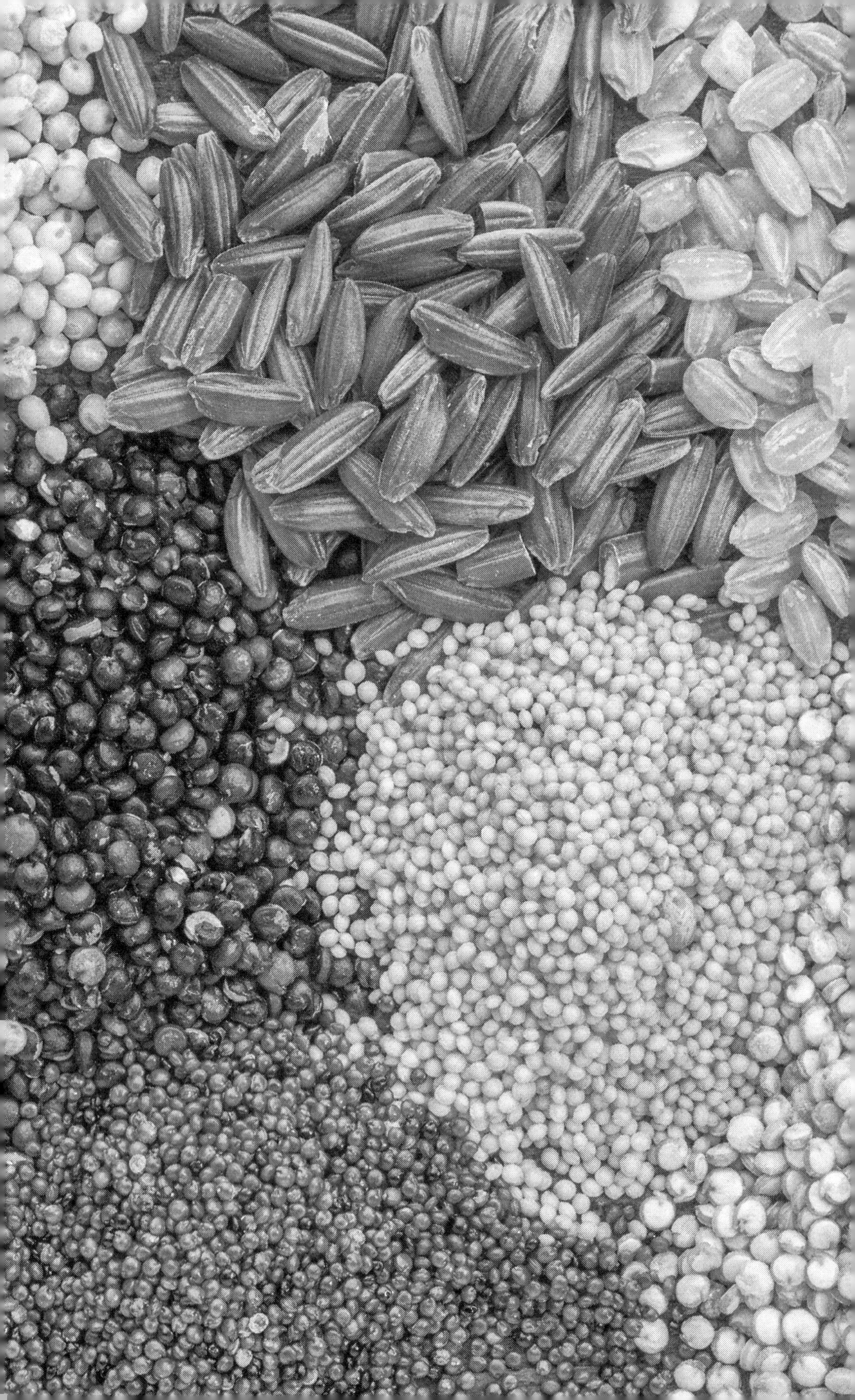

Basic Sautéed Greens
2 T. olive oil
1 head of kale, Swiss chard, collard greens, etc.
Salt and pepper to taste
Optional: crushed red pepper, lemon juice, garlic

1. Combine greens (removing stems).
2. Heat oil in a large pan over medium heat.
3. Add greens, salt, pepper and your choice of optional seasonings.
4. Stir until greens are softened and bright in color (2-5 minutes). You may add a little vegetable broth to wilt the thicker greens. Don't let them get mushy or turn gray. You will enjoy them most when they have a little 'crunch' to them!

Basic Beans

1 cup dried beans
2 cups water
Salt and pepper to taste
Optional: A small one inch square of kombu*

1. In a pot, bring the beans, water and kombu to a boil, then simmer. Depending on the size of the bean, it can take anywhere from 30 -90 minutes for the beans to get soft.
2. Drain and discard whatever is left of the kombu.
3. Season to taste with salt and pepper.

*Kombu is a form of sea vegetable found in the health food store. It is perfect to eliminate 'gas' from beans!

Basic Quinoa Bowl Example
Grain: ½–¾ cooked quinoa
Green: 1 handful raw Swiss chard, finely chopped
Bean: ½ cup cooked navy beans
Other vegetables: 1 chopped tomato
Dressing: extra virgin olive oil, apple cider vinegar, salt and pepper to taste

(cont.)

Combine ingredients in a bowl and serve warm or at room temperature. *Serves 1*

You can use any combination of greens, beans and vegetables that you like!

Basic Rice Bowl Example
Grain: ½–¾ cup cooked brown rice
Greens: 2 handfuls spinach
Bean: ½ cup cooked black beans
Dressing: salsa

Combine ingredients in a bowl and serve warm or at room temperature. *Serves 1*

Don't forget to experiment with different quantities depending on your hunger levels and different grain/bean/vegetable combinations.

SMOOTHIES

Add two scoops of protein powder, a handful of ice and blend all ingredients to make these protein drinks!
All smoothies serve 1.
NOTE: All ingredients are optional, choose the ones you like!

Simple Green Smoothies
1 cup 'base' (non-dairy milk of your choice or water)
½ cup fruit of choice (berries, apple, tropical fruit, etc.)
½ banana
Handful of spinach or kale
1 tsp. ground flaxseed
(Suggestion: Shaklee Vanilla Protein Powder)

Yam - Orange Smoothie
Yes, you read that right. If you make sweet potatoes or yams for dinner and you have any left over, throw them in your smoothie the next morning!
½ cup almond milk plus ½ cup orange juice
1 large yam or sweet potato, baked, peeled, and chopped
2 T. honey
(Suggestion: Shaklee Vanilla Protein Powder)

Sweet Sensation
1 cup cashew milk
1 apple, core removed
1 small pear, peeled and core removed
½ tsp. cinnamon
¼ tsp. fresh grated nutmeg
(Suggestion: Shaklee Vanilla Protein Powder)

The Elvis
1 cup almond milk
1 banana
1 T. nut butter
1 T. raw cacao powder
(Suggestion: Shaklee Chocolate Protein Powder)

Cherry Delight
1 cup almond milk
1 cup frozen cherries
½ cup plain non-dairy yogurt (non-GMO soy or almond)
¼ cup old-fashioned oats (use gluten-free oats)
½ tsp. vanilla extract
¼ tsp. almond extract
pinch of salt
(Suggestion: Shaklee Vanilla Protein Powder)

Strawberry Green Machine
1 cup non-dairy milk
½ cup frozen strawberries
½ cup frozen mango
Handful of baby spinach
(Suggestion: Shaklee Strawberry Protein Powder)

Morning Boost
1 cup coconut milk
1 large apple, cut into small pieces
½ frozen banana
1 handful of baby spinach
1 T. almond butter
1 T. ground flaxseed
½ tsp. cinnamon
(Suggestion: Shaklee Café Latte Protein Powder)

Hazelnut Chocolate Spice
1 cup almond milk
1 T. raw cacao powder
1 T. nut butter
1 cup spinach
10 hazelnuts
1 T. chia seeds
(Suggestion: Shaklee Chocolate Protein Powder)

Sweet Potato Pie
1 cup coconut milk
1 sweet potato, peeled, roasted and mashed
1 apple, cored and cut

(cont.)

¼ cup pecans
2 pitted medjool dates
¼ tsp. allspice
(Suggestion: Shaklee Café Latte Protein Powder)

Peanut Butter and Jelly
1 cup almond milk
1 T. almond butter
1 cup of frozen strawberries
(Suggestion: Shaklee Strawberry Protein Powder)

Peaches and Cream
1 cup unsweetened vanilla almond milk
1 cup frozen peach slices
½ tsp. cinnamon
(Suggestion: Shaklee Café Latte Protein Powder)

Blueberry Pancake
1 cup coconut milk 12q
1 cup blueberries
1–2 T. rolled oats
1 T. pure maple syrup
(Suggestion: Shaklee Vanilla Protein Powder)

Apple Pie
1 large red apple, cored
1 cup unsweetened almond milk
½ cup non-dairy yogurt
1 tsp. ground cinnamon
pinch of ground nutmeg
pinch of ground ginger
tiny pinch of ground cloves
(Suggestion: Shaklee Vanilla Protein Powder)

Coconut Cream
1 cup coconut milk
½ frozen banana
1 T. coconut oil, melted
1 T. unsweetened coconut flakes + additional for topping
(Suggestion: Shaklee Vanilla Protein Powder)

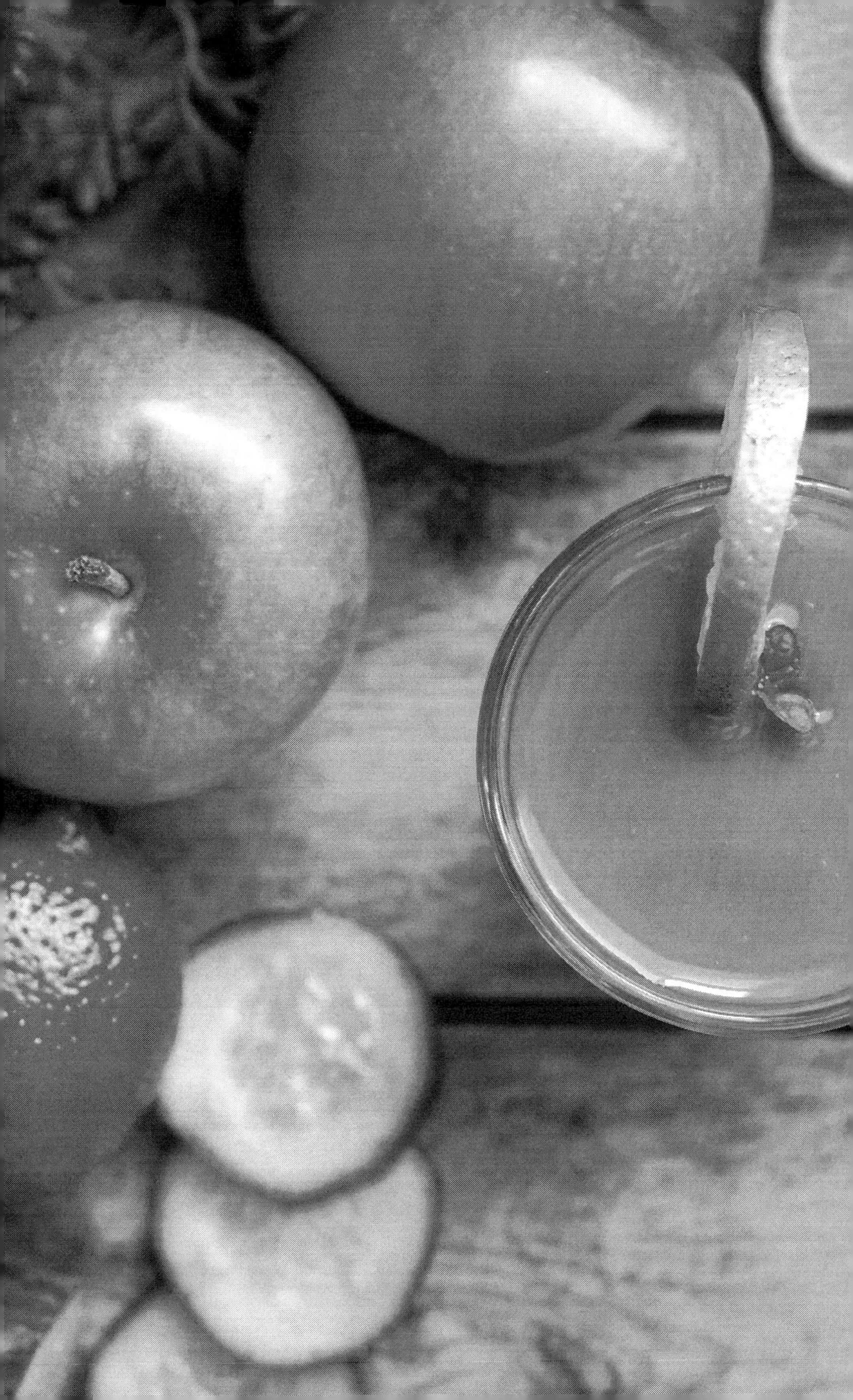

BREAKFASTS

Brown Rice Porridge

Use leftover brown rice to make a satisfying breakfast.

1 cup cooked brown rice
1 cup coconut or almond milk
2 T. dried fruit of your choice (I like dried cherries or blueberries)
Dash cinnamon
1 T. honey
1 egg
¼ tsp. vanilla extract
1 T. butter

1. Combine rice, milk, dried fruit, cinnamon, and honey in a small saucepan.
2. Bring to a boil, then reduce heat to low and simmer 20 minutes.
3. Beat egg in a small bowl.
4. Temper the egg by whisking some of the hot rice into the egg mixture a tablespoon at a time until you have incorporated about 6 tablespoons.
5. Stir the egg into the rice along with the vanilla and butter and continue cooking for 1–2 minutes until thickened. *Serves 1*

Alyson's Mediterranean Breakfast

This is a common breakfast at my house. If you are not a fan of sardines, I encourage you to experiment. There are varieties that come in olive oil, tomato sauce, lemon juice etc. Sardines are exceptionally good for you and a great source of calcium; bones and all!

1 small can of sardines, drained
1 small tomato, sliced
A few slices of cucumber
A few slices of feta or goat cheese

½ cup of a fruit of your choice (I like grapes with this)
Rice crackers or a rice cake

Arrange everything on a plate and enjoy with a cup of tea.
Serves 1

Homemade Granola
This is for the adventurous. If you don't feel like making your own, find a healthy granola that is low in all natural sugar content.

2 ¼ cups quick-cooking oats
1 cup sunflower seeds
1 cup raisins
¾ cup dried goji berries, coarsely chopped
½ cup pitted dates
½ cup raw green pumpkin seeds, coarsely chopped
1 tsp. ground cinnamon
½ tsp. ground ginger

1. Combine all ingredients in a bowl and toss to combine.
2. Store in an airtight container for up to 3 weeks. You can use any combination of nuts, seeds or dried fruit that you enjoy.

Serves 12 (Makes enough for a family.)

Tip: To serve warm, combine ½ cup granola with ½ cup liquid (unsweetened hemp milk, unsweetened soymilk or water work well) and simmer on the stovetop until oats are softened, 1 to 2 minutes.

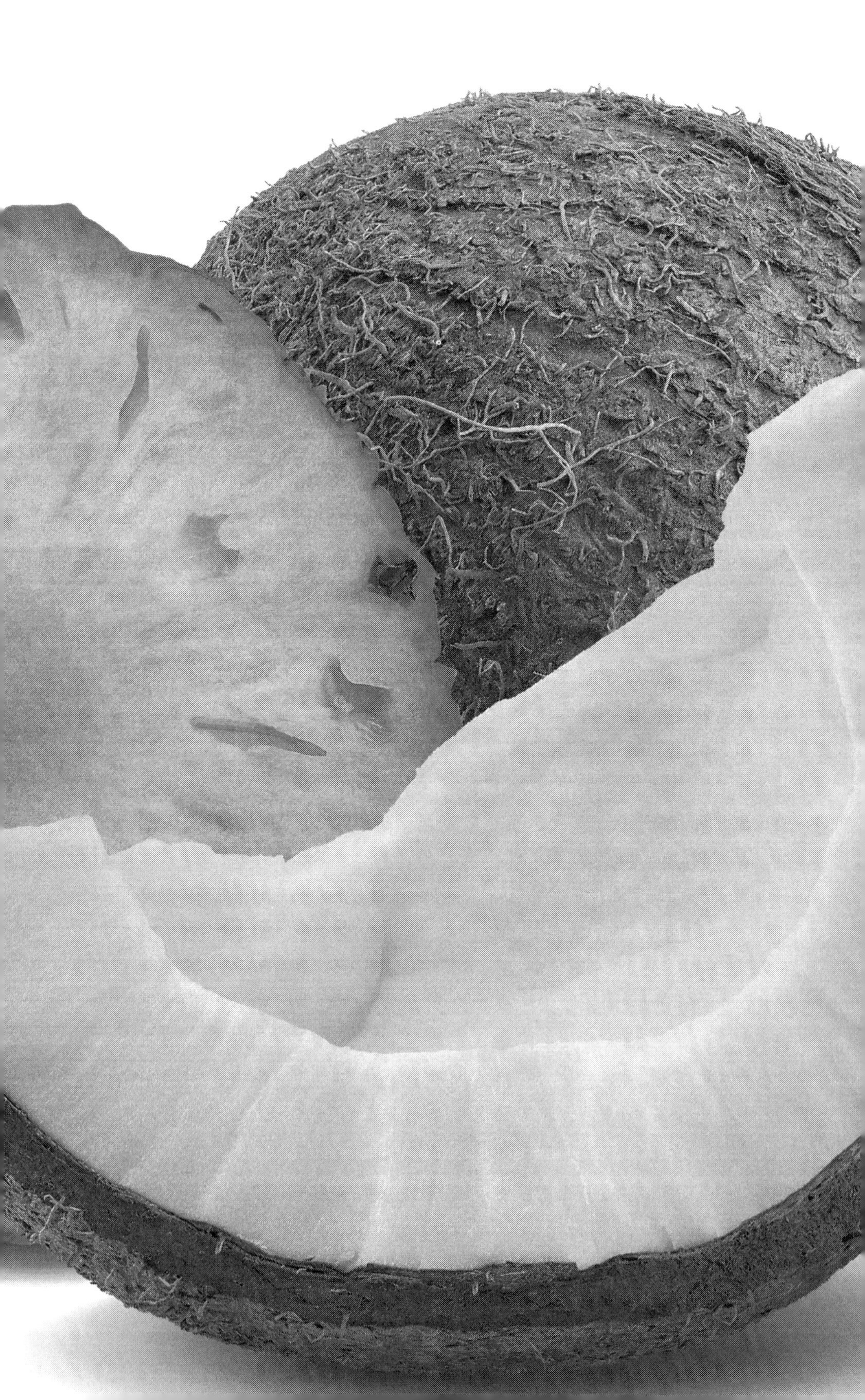

Pineapple Coconut Yogurt

1 cup fresh pineapple chunks, diced small (or use half of a 15 oz. can crushed pineapple, drained)
1 container of coconut yogurt or your choice of plain non-dairy yogurt
¼ cup your choice of nuts (my suggestion is macadamia nuts)
Optional: toasted coconut

Open yogurt, sprinkle pineapple and coconut (if using) over yogurt. *Serves 1*

Optional: To toast coconut, spread flaked unsweetened coconut on aluminum foil and toast in toaster oven until golden (about 30 seconds).

Easy Flax Breakfast Pudding

This "pudding" can be put together in the microwave in 3–4 minutes. You can add berries or other "mix-ins" - see suggestions below. The flax gives it lots of fiber and good fat, plus a nice nutty flavor.

¼ cup flaxseed meal (or ground flaxseed)
¼ cup water
1 egg
1 T. honey or agave syrup
Mix-ins as desired (see below)

1. Mix flaxseed meal, egg, and water in a microwave-safe bowl.
2. Microwave on high for about 45 seconds.
3. Move the cooked part of the pudding towards the center of the bowl and add any mix-ins you want.
4. Microwave for about 45-60 more seconds, depending on mix-ins.
5. Stir and eat. *Serves 1*

Possible Additions:
Fresh berries or other fruit
Unsweetened coconut
Peanut butter or other nut butters *(cont.)*

Maple syrup
"Healthy" jam (one that does not contain refined sugar)
Chopped nuts

Black Bean Breakfast Burrito
1 or 2 egg whites
¼ cup canned black beans, rinsed and drained
2 T. salsa
2 T. diced goat cheese
1 small whole-wheat tortilla

1. Scramble eggs, beans, salsa and cheese.
2. Cook over low heat until consistency you like.
3. Fill tortilla with egg mixture. *Serves 1*

Morning Glory Muffins
Organic nonstick cooking spray
1 ¼ cups all-purpose flour (spooned and leveled)
½ cup packed organic dark-brown sugar (or natural sweetener alternative)
½ tsp. baking soda
½ tsp. baking powder
½ tsp. ground nutmeg
½ tsp. sea salt
1 cup old-fashioned rolled oats
½ cup raisins
3 T. extra-virgin olive oil
1 large egg
1/3 cup non-dairy milk
4 medium carrots, shredded (I buy the bag of already shredded carrots!)
1 medium ripe banana, mashed

1. Preheat oven to 400°F.
2. Coat a 12-cup muffin pan with cooking spray.
3. In a large bowl, whisk together flour, brown sugar, baking soda, baking powder, nutmeg, and salt until there are no lumps.
4. Stir in oats and raisins.
5. Add oil, egg, milk, carrots, and banana and stir until blended

6. Fill each muffin cup with ¼ cup batter.
7. Bake until a toothpick inserted in center of a muffin comes out clean, 23 to 25 minutes.
8. Serve muffins warm or at room temperature. *Makes 12*

NOTE: To store, keep in an airtight container up to 3 days.

Simple Buckwheat Porridge

1 cup water
½ cup buckwheat groats
¼ tsp. salt
1 T. maple syrup
¼ tsp. cinnamon
½ tsp. vanilla extract
2 T. soy creamer or soy milk (almond or hemp will also work)

Optional add-ins once cooked: raisins, chopped dates, flax or chia seeds, a spoonful of almond butter, sliced banana, raw pistachios, a few sliced peaches (frozen or fresh) and any other fruits and nuts are welcome!

1. Add the water and groats to a soup pot.
2. Add in the salt, cinnamon, maple syrup and vanilla. Bring to a boil and then cover with lid and reduce to a simmer.
3. Allow groats to simmer for at least ten minutes – check the texture of the groats; they should be squishy, but not mushy or too watery.
4. Once the groats are tender with all the water absorbed, add in the soy milk or creamer and continue to simmer with the lid off.
5. Add in the chia seeds, flax seeds and dried fruit – and anything else that you want to melt into the porridge. A spoonful of vegan buttery spread is also nice.
6. Simmer until nice and thick. Then turn off heat. Allow the groats to cool and thicken about ten minutes before serving.
7. Serve with fresh or thawed fruit, another splash of soy milk and some optional spices and nuts on top. *Serves 2*

Superfood Cereal

2 T. raw cacao nibs
2 T. unsweetened coconut flakes
1 T. chia seeds
2 T. sliced almonds
1 T. hemp seeds
3 T. fresh blueberries
1 cup unsweetened almond milk
Stevia to taste if needed

1. Place a cereal-sized bowl on the counter and add dry ingredients, except blueberries.
2. Add unsweetened almond milk and a few drops of stevia.
3. Let soak for 5 minutes, top with blueberries and enjoy! *Serves 1*

Apple Raisin Quinoa

1–2 cups cooked quinoa
½ cup water (enough to create a porridge consistency)
1 apple, chopped
¼ cup raisins
1 tsp. cinnamon

1. In a small pot, combine all ingredients.
2. Bring to a boil, and then reduce to simmer until water is absorbed, about 5 minutes. *Serves 2*

Japanese Style Rice Porridge

1–2 cups cooked brown rice
½ cup water (enough to create a porridge consistency)
1 T. soy sauce
½ sheet nori (seaweed used with sushi, found in the health food store) cut with scissors into strips
1 T. sesame seeds

1. Combine rice and water in a small pot.
2. Bring to a boil, and then simmer until water is absorbed, about 5 minutes.
3. Mix in soy sauce and top with nori and sesame seeds. *Serves 2*

DRESSINGS

You can use dressings over basic greens, grains or salads (whisk ingredients together, shake them together in a jar or blend in a mini-processor or blender).

Most Natural Asian Dressing
¼ cup extra virgin olive oil
3 T. apple cider vinegar
4 T. tahini
1 T. Tamari soy sauce

Basic Vinaigrette
1 cup extra virgin olive oil
¾ cup vinegar of your choice or lemon juice
1 large garlic clove, minced
½ tsp. salt
Dried or fresh herbs to taste

Fresh Creamy Dressing
½ cup lemon juice
3 T. melted coconut oil
2 T. umeboshi plum vinegar
2 cups loosely packed fresh basil
1 tsp. salt
1 tsp. ground ginger
1 tsp. garlic powder

Cranberry Vinaigrette
3 T. red wine vinegar
1/3 cup olive oil
¼ cup fresh cranberries
1 T. Dijon mustard
½ tsp. minced garlic
½ tsp. salt
½ tsp. ground black pepper
2 T. water

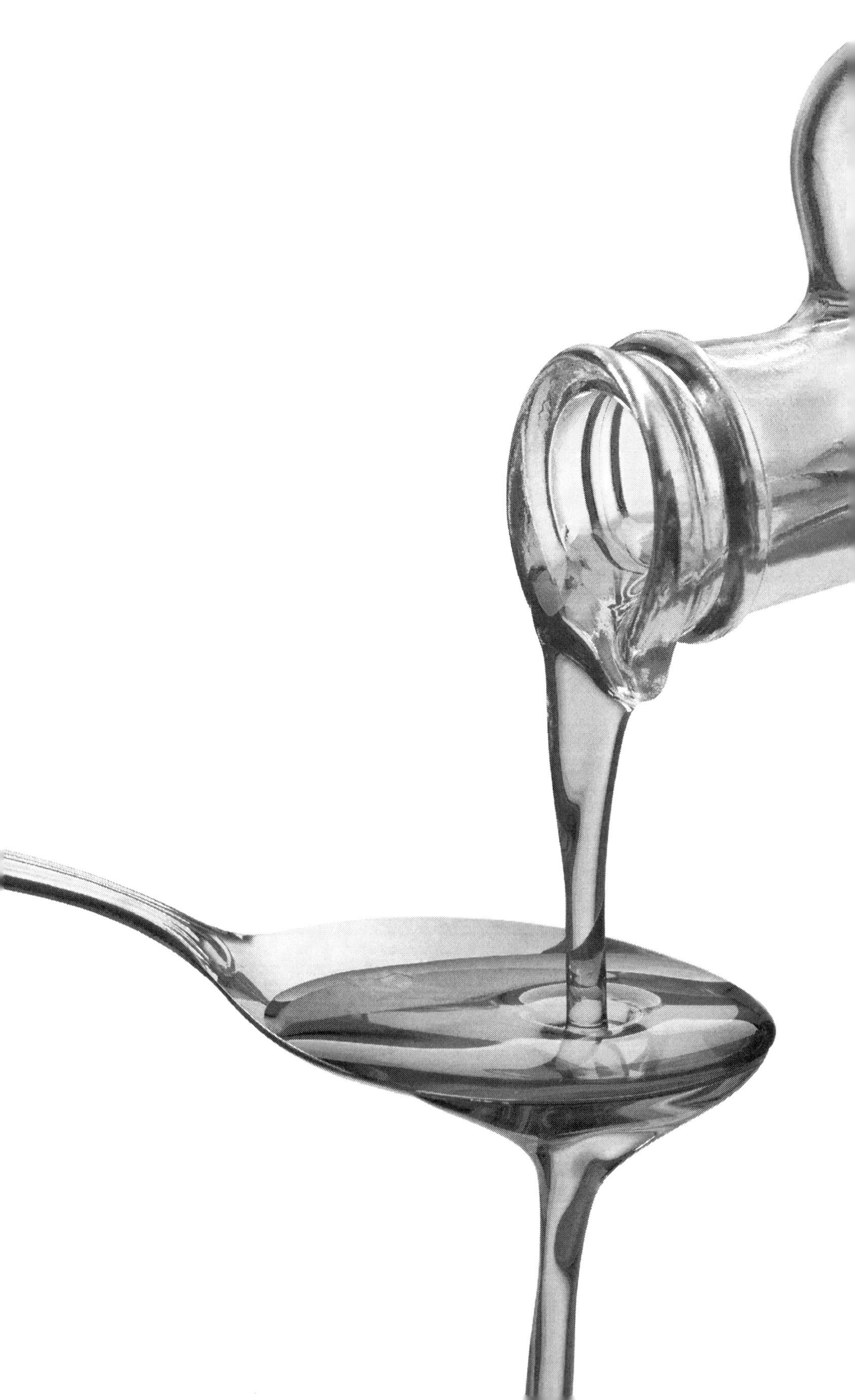

SALADS

Warm Spinach Salad with Tuna

6 cups baby spinach
1 can tuna packed in water
1 T. extra virgin olive oil
1 tsp. lemon juice
1 medium clove garlic, minced
Sea salt and pepper to taste

1. Combine oil, lemon juice, garlic, salt and pepper to taste in a saucepan and heat until warm.
2. Drizzle over spinach leaves and top with tuna.
   Serves 1

Tabouli Salad

1 cup quinoa (rinsed)
½ medium red onion, minced
2 cloves garlic, press or chopped
3 cups minced fresh parsley
1 medium tomato, chopped
3 T. extra virgin olive oil
1 T. fresh lemon juice or wine vinegar
Sea salt and pepper to taste

1. Cook quinoa according to package directions.
2. Let cool.
3. Combine all ingredients and mix well.

For added flavor, add more olive oil and lemon juice. Serves 4

Bean Salad

2 tsp. olive oil
1 tsp. dried oregano
2 cloves of crushed garlic
¼ cup apple cider vinegar
3 x 16 oz. cans beans - red, black, and chickpeas
1 cup diced tomatoes (or more if you want)
½ cup sweet onion (or less if you want)
1/3 cup chopped parsley *(cont.)*

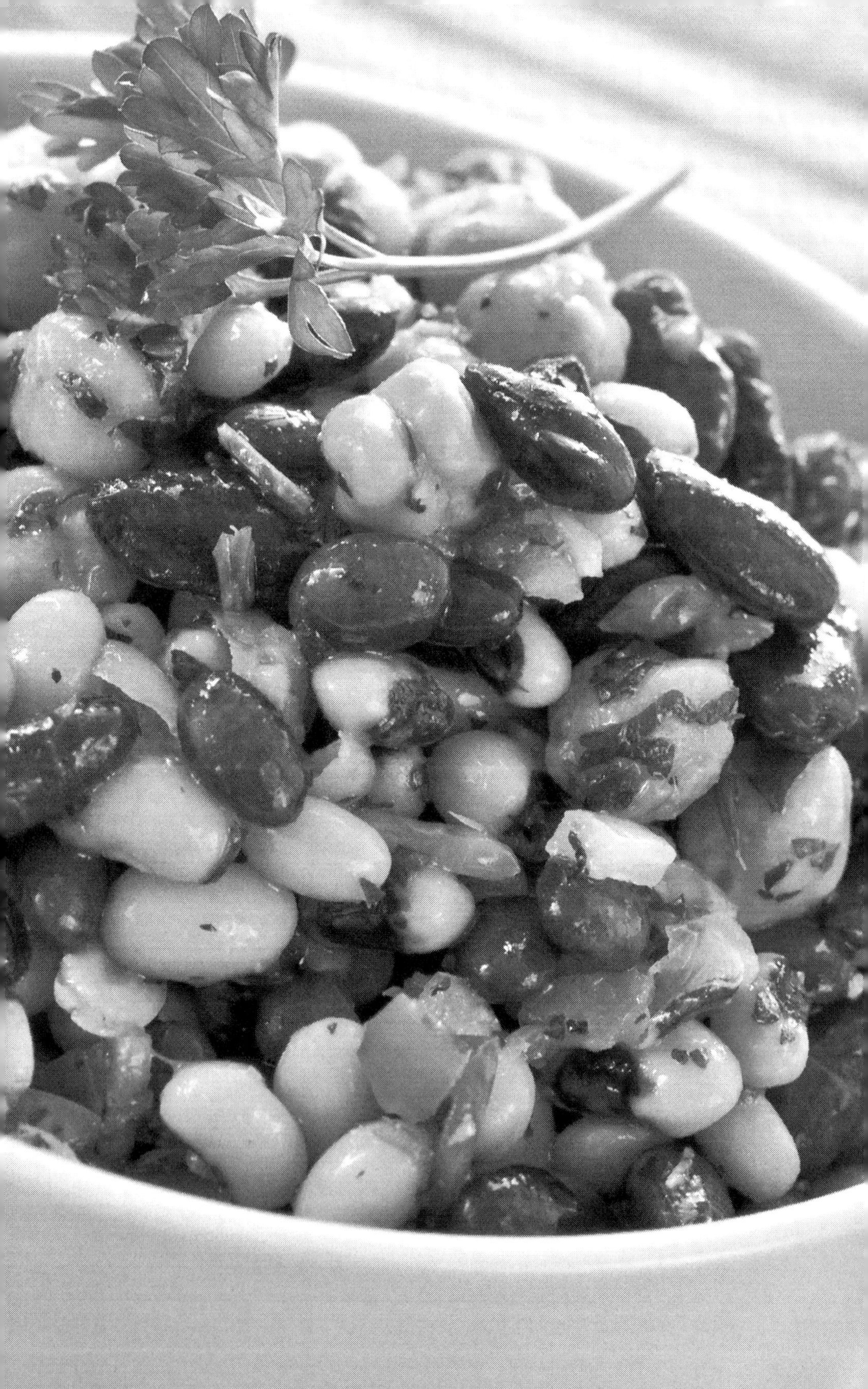

½ tsp. salt
½ tsp. pepper

1. Sauté 1 tsp. olive oil with oregano and crushed garlic for 30 sec.
2. Add vinegar and remove from heat.
3. Combine liquid with the rinsed and drained canned beans in a bowl.
4. Chill for 30 min.
5. After this has chilled add 1 tsp. olive oil, tomato, and next 4 ingredients and serve. *Serves 4*

Warm Lentil, Grape, Mint and Feta Salad
3 T. extra virgin olive oil
2 leeks, white and green parts, sliced thin
2 T. rice wine vinegar
2 tsp. organic mustard
2 cups cooked lentils (green lentils work best)
1 ½ cups red grapes, halved
¼ cup chopped roasted pistachios
3 T. fresh mint, finely chopped
3 T. parsley, finely chopped
¼ cup crumbled feta

1. Heat oil in skillet over medium heat.
2. Add leeks and sauté for 7-9 minutes or until tender and translucent.
3. Remove from heat and stir in vinegar and mustard.
4. Combine lentils, leek mixture, grapes, pistachios, mint and parsley in a large bowl.
5. Season with salt and pepper, if desired and top with crumbled feta. *Serves 4*

Chickpea and Raisin Salad
½ cup raisins
¼ cup red wine vinegar
2 tsp. honey
2 x 15.5 oz. cans chickpeas, rinsed
½ cup fresh cilantro or flat-leaf parsley leaves
2 scallions, thinly sliced
¼ cup olive oil *(cont.)*

¼ tsp. ground cumin
Sea salt and black pepper

1. In a small saucepan, combine the raisins, vinegar and honey and bring just to a simmer.
2. Remove from heat and let cool.
3. In a large bowl, toss the chickpeas, cilantro, scallions, and raisin mixture with the oil, cumin, salt and pepper. Enjoy. *Serves 4*

Beet, Carrot and Pear Salad
1 raw beet, scrubbed and peeled
1 pear
2 carrots, peeled
A couple of handfuls of salad greens
½ cup walnuts, chopped
¼ cup raisins

1. Grate the beet, pear and carrots by hand or put through a food processor.
2. Combine with the greens, walnuts and raisins.
3. Toss with Most Natural Dressing. *Serves 2*

Red Cabbage and Grapefruit Salad
Salad:
4 cups thinly sliced red cabbage
2 cups segmented grapefruit (seeds, peel, and pith removed)
3 T. dried cranberries
2 T. pumpkin seeds

Dressing:
2-3 T. lemon juice
A pinch of salt
A pinch of black pepper

1. Place salad ingredients in a large mixing bowl.
2. Add dressing ingredients and toss to mix.

Salad will keep for 2 to 3 days in the fridge. Serves 4

Green Bean Slaw

½ lb. haricots vert (thin green beans)
2 T. extra-virgin olive oil
1 garlic clove, minced
½ small red onion, thinly sliced
¼ cup plus 1 T. cider vinegar
2 ½ T. water
1 ½ tsp. Dijon mustard
1 ½ tsp. honey
¼ tsp. celery seeds
Worcestershire sauce
Hot sauce
Salt and freshly ground black pepper
Optional: 1 hard-cooked egg, chopped, for garnish

1. In a large pot of boiling salted water, cook the beans until crisp-tender, about 2 minutes.
2. Drain, rinse and pat dry.
3. In a large skillet, heat the olive oil.
4. Add the onion and garlic and cook over moderate heat until fragrant, about 3 minutes.
5. Stir in the vinegar, water, mustard, honey and celery seeds.
6. Transfer to a large bowl.
7. Add the beans and toss well.
8. Add a few dashes of Worcestershire sauce and hot sauce and season with salt and pepper. Garnish the slaw with the chopped egg and serve warm or at room temperature. *Serves 4*

Mediterranean Lentil Salad

¾ cup dried green lentils
(You want to end up with 2 cups cooked)
2 cups water
3 oz. canned/jar roasted red peppers, chopped
2 T. finely minced onion
2 medium cloves garlic, pressed
½ cup chopped fresh basil
⅓ cup coarsely chopped walnuts
3 T. balsamic vinegar
1 T. fresh lemon juice *(cont.)*

2 T. + 2 T. extra virgin olive oil
Salt and pepper to taste
1 bunch arugula, chopped

1. Wash lentils, remove any foreign matter, and drain.
2. Combine lentils and 2 cups lightly salted water in medium saucepan. Bring to a boil.
3. Reduce heat, and cook at low temperature for about 20 minutes, or until lentils are cooked but still firm. Cook gently so lentils don't get mushy.
4. When done, drain any excess water, and lightly rinse under cold water. Continue to drain excess water.
5. Mince onion and press garlic.
6. Place lentils in a bowl and add peppers, onion, garlic, basil, walnuts, vinegar, and 2 T. olive oil. Season with salt and pepper to taste.
7. Marinate for at least 1 hour before serving.
8. Toss arugula with 2 T. olive oil, 1 T. lemon juice, salt and pepper. Serve on plate with lentils. *Serves 4*

Sweet Potato Salad with Orange-Maple Dressing

This salad can remain at room temperature up to two hours before serving.

Dressing:
¼ cup extra-virgin olive oil
2 tsp. pure maple syrup
2 tsp. orange juice
2 tsp. sherry wine vinegar or balsamic vinegar
1 tsp. fresh lemon juice
2 tsp. minced peeled fresh ginger
½ tsp. ground cinnamon
¼ tsp. ground nutmeg

Salad:
3 lb. red-skinned sweet potatoes (yams), peeled, cut into ¾ inch cubes
½ cup green onions, chopped
½ cup fresh parsley, chopped
½ cup pecans, toasted, coarsely chopped
¼ cup golden raisins

¼ cup brown raisins

1. For dressing, whisk all ingredients to blend in small bowl and season to taste with salt and pepper.
2. For salad, steam sweet potatoes in batches until potatoes are just tender, about 10 minutes per batch and then transfer them to a large bowl.
3. Cool to room temperature.
4. Add green onions, parsley, pecans and all raisins.
5. Pour dressing over and toss gently to blend.
6. Season salad to taste with salt and pepper.
7. Let stand at room temperature. *Serves 6*

Quinoa Salad with Black Beans and Toasted Cumin Seeds

2 cups cooked quinoa
2 tsp. cumin seeds
1 cup finely diced plum tomatoes (about 4)
3 T. freshly squeezed lime juice (3 to 4 limes)
2 tsp. raw agave nectar
1 tsp. extra virgin olive oil
1 x 15 oz. can black beans, drained and rinsed
1 cup finely chopped scallions
¼ tsp. salt
Mixed greens, for serving

1. Place quinoa in a large mixing bowl, if it isn't already cooling in one.
2. To toast cumin seeds, preheat an
3. 8-inch pan over low heat. Place cumin seeds in dry pan and toss often for about 5 minutes.
4. Immediately transfer to a medium-size mixing bowl. Add tomatoes, lime juice, agave and oil to mixing bowl and mix well.
5. When quinoa is cooled, mix it in.
6. Fold in beans and scallions. Taste for salt.
7. You can serve immediately or let sit for a bit for the flavors to meld.
8. Serve over mixed greens. *Serves 4*

Kale Salad (RAW)
1 bunch of kale, shredded (discard the woody stems)
1 cup tomatoes, diced
1 cup avocado
2 ½ T. olive oil
1 ½ T. lemon juice
1 tsp. sea salt
½ tsp. cayenne pepper

Using your hands, toss the ingredients together, squeezing to cream the avocado. *Serves 4*

Hint: The more avocado you use, the richer and creamier (and, frankly, tastier) this salad gets.

Arugula Salad with Walnut Croutons
½ medium yellow onion, thinly sliced
1 cup hot water
2 T. light vinegar
1 bunch arugula

Dressing:
2 medium cloves garlic, pressed
2 T. chopped fresh parsley
1 T. fresh lemon juice
1 T. extra virgin olive oil
Sea salt and black pepper to taste
½ cup coarsely chopped walnuts
2 oz. feta cheese (optional)

1. Press garlic and let sit for 5 minutes.
2. Slice onion thin and soak in hot water and vinegar while preparing rest of salad.
3. Whisk together the dressing ingredients, adding olive oil at the end, a little at a time.
4. Wash and dry arugula.
5. Squeeze out excess liquid from onions.
6. Combine onions and arugula and toss with dressing.
7. Sprinkle salad with walnuts just before serving.
8. Top with cheese (optional). *Serves 2*

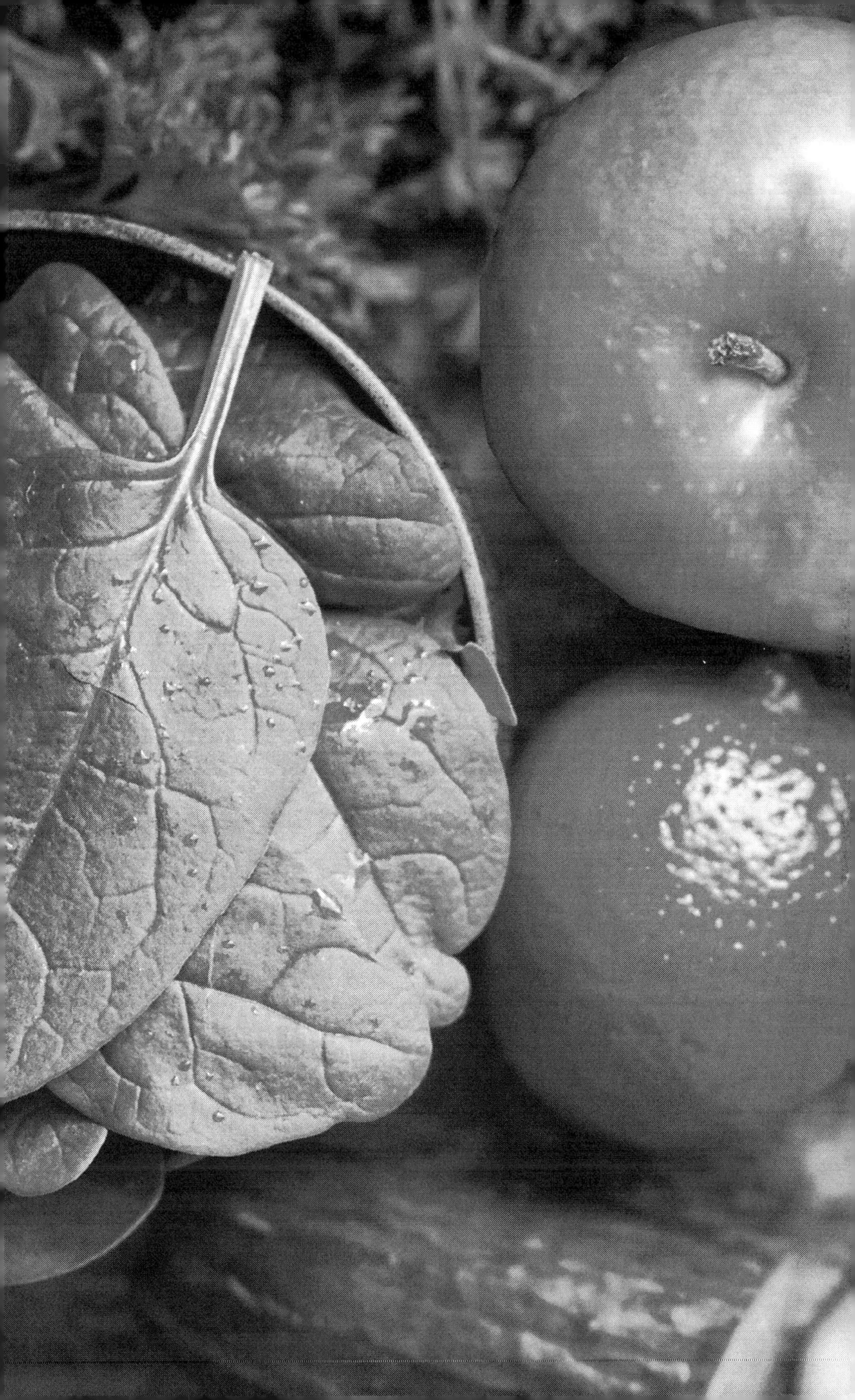

Spinach Beet Berry Salad (RAW)
Handful of baby spinach
1 small beet, shredded
1 small carrot, shredded
½ red pepper, cut in chunks
¼ cup red onion, cut in chunks
Sprinkle of raw slivered almonds
6 or more ripe juicy strawberries, sliced
Black olives (optional)

Honey Dressing:
½ cup extra virgin olive oil
3 T. fresh lemon juice
1 tsp. Dijon mustard
2 T. honey
2 T. water
Optional: Sea salt

Layer the ingredients into a big salad bowl and drizzle with honey dressing. *Serves 2*

Fruited Celery Salad (RAW)
1 cup celery, cut on a diagonal
1 orange, peeled, seeded and sectioned (please grate ½ tsp. zest before peeling for dressing)
1 medium apple, unpeeled, thinly sliced
½ fresh pineapple, cored, cut into cubes; if using canned, drain juice
Lettuce leaves

Dressing:
2 T. lime juice
1 T. honey
2 tsp. water
½ tsp. poppy seeds
½ tsp. grated orange peel

1. Place all ingredients in a jar and shake well.
2. In a medium bowl, mix all salad ingredients except lettuce.

3. Pour dressing over salad, toss lightly to coat. Cover and refrigerate.
4. Serve on lettuce lined plates.

Asian Cabbage and Peanut Salad (RAW)
2 cups Napa cabbage, thinly sliced or shredded
2 cups curly kale, thinly sliced or shredded
2 cups carrots, shredded
1 cup raw peanuts

Dressing:
¼ cup sesame oil
¼ cup lime or lemon juice
2 T. rice wine vinegar
1 T. Tamari soy sauce
½ T. honey

1. Combine veggies in a bowl.
2. Mix together dressing ingredients in a jar and shake well.
3. Pour dressing over veggies and toss well to combine.
4. Let sit for 20-30 minutes.
5. Mix in peanuts and serve. *Serves 4*

Garlic Shrimp Salad
4 medium cloves garlic, minced
1 lb. medium-sized cooked shrimp, best bought still frozen
1 bunch asparagus, cut into 1-inch pieces, discarding bottom fourth
3 T. vegetable broth
1 fresh tomato, diced into ½-inch pieces
3 T. fresh parsley, chopped (or 3 tsp. dried parsley if fresh not available)
Small head of romaine lettuce, chopped
Salt and fresh cracked black pepper to taste
Optional: 2 oz. crumbled goat cheese

Dressing:
3 T. fresh lemon juice
2 T. extra virgin olive oil
1 T. Dijon mustard
1 tsp. honey

(cont.)

Salt and pepper to taste

1. Make sure shrimp is completely thawed and patted dry with a paper towel, or it will dilute the flavor of the salad.
2. Add broth to medium skillet and after it has heated up, sauté asparagus for 5 minutes.
3. Whisk together lemon, oil, mustard, honey, garlic, salt and pepper.
4. Toss shrimp, asparagus, parsley, and tomato with dressing and herbs. Allow shrimp salad to marinate for at least 15 minutes.
5. Discard outer leaves of lettuce head, rinse, dry, and chop.
6. Serve shrimp mixture on bed of lettuce and top with crumbled goat cheese, if desired. *Serves 4*

Dynasty Salad
1–2 handfuls spinach, torn
1 cup Napa cabbage
Carrots/cucumbers/bean sprouts/snap peas
Fresh mint and basil leaves
Sesame seeds, toasted
½ cup cooked mung beans
(Use Asian Essence Dressing)

1. Combine all ingredients in a large bowl. Make it big and beautiful! It's all good for you!
2. Toss well with the dressing to combine. *Serves 2*

Spinach and Persimmon Salad with Parsley Mustard Dressing
4 cups baby spinach
1 persimmon, cut into cubes
2 baby leeks, thinly sliced
½ cup white beans, drained and rinsed
¼ cup pine nuts or sliced almonds

1. Mix all ingredients in a bowl and dress.

Dressing:
3 T. apple cider vinegar
½ cup olive oil

2 cloves garlic, minced
1 T. whole grain mustard
2 T. chopped parsley
Salt and pepper to taste

1. Whisk all ingredients together and dress your salad.

Serves 2

Herbed Watermelon Salad with Cherry Tomatoes, Feta, and Toasted Pepitas

4 cups cubed watermelon
2 cups halved cherry tomatoes
¾ cup crumbled feta
1/3 cup minced herbs (I use a combination of mint, basil, and oregano)
¼ cup olive oil, divided
¼ cup raw, hulled pepitas (pumpkin seeds)
2 T. fresh squeezed lemon juice
Sea salt and fresh ground black pepper to taste

1. Prep the watermelon, cherry tomatoes, herbs, and feta, and combine in a large serving bowl.
2. Make the vinaigrette by whisking the lemon juice and a pinch of sea salt into 3 tablespoons olive oil. Drizzle over the watermelon mixture.
3. Toast the pepitas by heating a small skillet over medium heat. Add 1 T. olive oil and then toss in the pepitas. Stir gently and cook just until pepitas begin to pop. Toss toasted pepitas with a pinch of sea salt.
4. Sprinkle the warm pepitas over the salad, add a bit more dressing if needed, and serve.
   Serves 4-6

Coconut Lime Rice Salad

1 cup jasmine rice, uncooked
½ cup unsweetened, shredded coconut, toasted
¼ cup sliced almonds, toasted
2 limes, zested and juiced
1 small shallot, minced (about 2 T.)
2 T. rice wine vinegar
3-4 T. olive oil

(cont.)

Big pinch of sea salt

1. Cook the rice according to the package directions.
2. Allow rice to rest, covered, for at least 5 minutes. Scrape the rice into a large mixing bowl and fluff gently with a fork. Set aside.
3. To toast the coconut and almonds, preheat the oven to 350°F and spread the coconut and almonds on a single layer on a baking sheet. Toast for about 4 minutes, stirring after the first 2 minutes. (Watch the coconut and nuts carefully). Once cooled, toss with the lime zest and set aside.
4. In a small jar combine the lime juice (about 1 T. total), minced shallot, vinegar, olive oil, and a big pinch of sea salt. Fasten the lid on the jar and shake vigorously to combine. Pour the vinaigrette over the rice and fold gently with a spatula to combine. Add the coconut/almond/lime zest mixture and fold in gently to combine. Serve warm, room temperature, or chilled. Serves 4

Asparagus Ribbon Salad with Dried Cherries

1/3 cup dried cherries
1 small shallot, minced
3 T. olive oil
2 T. fresh-squeezed lemon juice
1 tsp. rice wine vinegar
½ tsp. sea salt
1 pound asparagus, washed

1. In a small bowl, whisk the lemon juice and vinegar into the olive oil. Add the sea salt, shallot and dried cherries. Set aside. The cherries will plump up while they steep in the vinaigrette.
2. To shave the asparagus, hold each stalk by the woody stem and use a peeler to shave upwards.
   Place shavings in a bowl, drizzle with the vinaigrette and toss. Check the salt and acid levels for taste and adjust as needed. If you have the time, cover and refrigerate for an hour or so. Serve cold. *Serves 4 as a side*

Grapefruit Arugula Salad
1 pink grapefruit
1 large bunch of arugula (about 4 cups)
1 bunch watercress (about 2 cups)
2 T. chopped walnuts

Dressing:
2 T. lemon juice
2 tsp. honey
2 tsp. Dijon mustard
1 T. extra virgin olive oil
Salt and pepper to taste

1. Peel the grapefruit and cut out each section between the membranes.
2. Prepare the arugula by tearing it to pieces, washing and drying.
3. Cut the tops of the watercress and spin dry with the arugula. A salad spinner is the best tool!
4. Mix together the dressing ingredients, toss with the salad greens and sections of grapefruit.
5. Top with chopped walnuts. *Serves 2*

Mediterranean Quinoa Salad
1 cup quinoa, rinsed
1 small cucumber, finely chopped
½ red onion, finely chopped
1 cup black olives (no pits)
½ yellow pepper, finely chopped
½ red pepper, finely chopped
1/3 cup extra virgin olive oil
2 T. red wine vinegar
Juice from ½ a lemon
1 tsp. sea salt
½ tsp. cracked black pepper
5 ounces cubed feta, crumbled
½ cup thinly sliced fresh basil

(cont.)

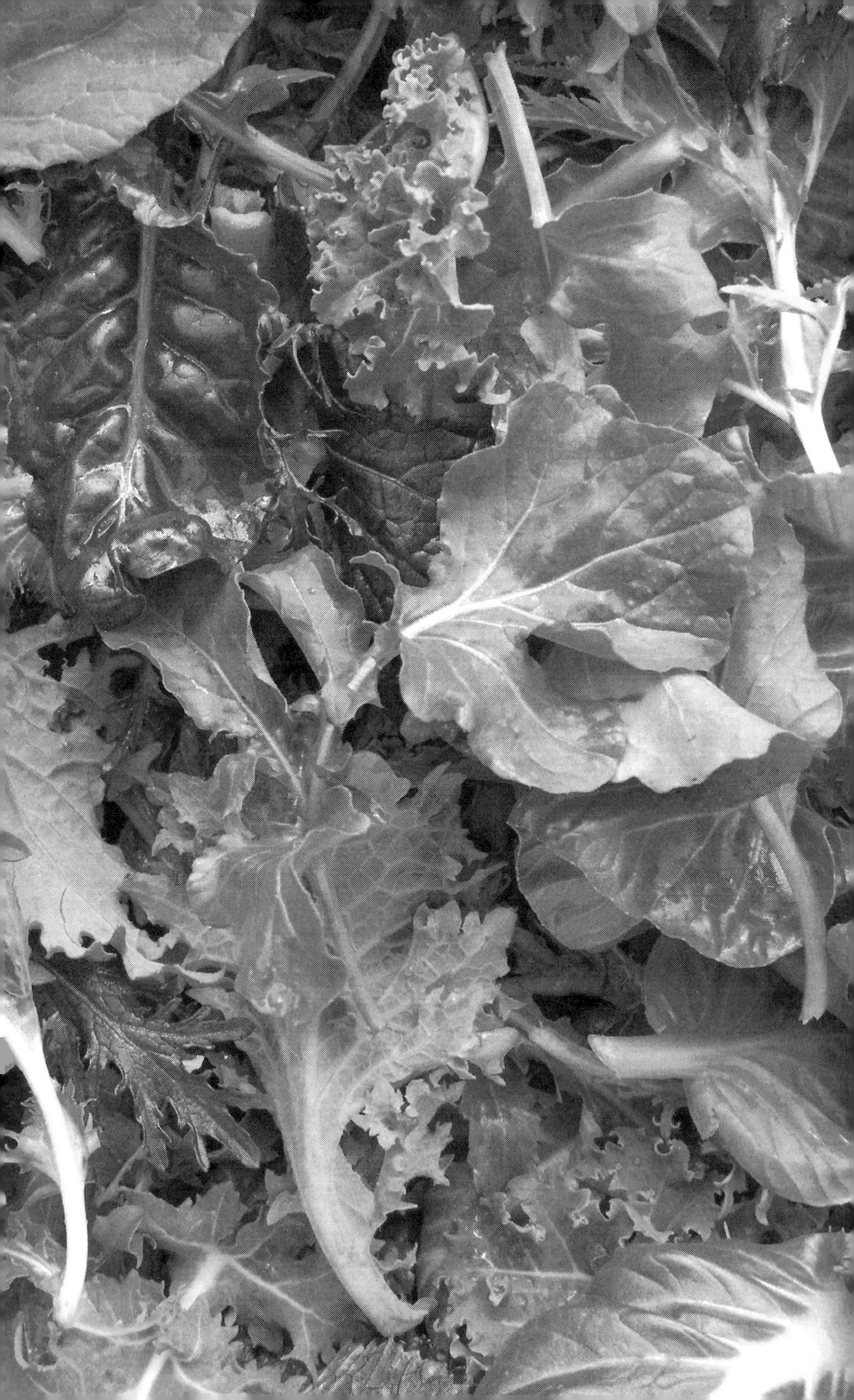

1. Cook the quinoa according to directions and drain completely.
2. Add the quinoa to a bowl and toss in the cucumber, onion, olives, and peppers.
3. Whisk together the olive oil, vinegar, lemon juice, salt, and pepper and drizzle it into the quinoa, tossing as you go. Then, toss in the feta and basil.
   Serve warm, room temperature, or chilled from the fridge. *Serves 4*

Creamy Honey Dijon Sala Dressing
1 avocado
¼ cup olive oil
3-5 T. water (depends on how thin you want your dressing)
2 T. lemon juice
1 T. dijon mustard
1 T. ginger
2 medjool dates, pitted
¼ tsp. Herbamare spice mix

Salad
2 cups romaine lettuce
½ fresh pear, sliced
2 medjool dates, pitted and chopped
Handful of walnuts
Yummy Croutons (Yes, I said Croutons!!! – Recipe below)

1. To make the dressing: combine all ingredients in a blender or food processor and process until smooth.
2. To make the salad: combine all ingredients in a bowl, add 2-3 T. dressing and toss until combined.
3. Serve topped with Yummy Croutons.

Yummy Croutons
6 pieces of gluten-free bread, cubed
2 T. ground flax seed
2 T. coconut oil, melted
2 T. fresh squeezed lemon juice
1 T. chia seeds
1 T. hemp seed
½ tsp. fresh parsley

(cont.)

¼ tsp. sage
½ tsp. rosemary
¼ tsp. basil
¼ tsp. oregano
¼ tsp. garlic powder
¼ tsp. Herbamare

1. Preheat oven to 375°F and line a cookie sheet with parchment paper or a silicon baking mat. Set aside.
2. Combine all ingredients but bread cubes in a small dish.
3. In a large bowl, add bread cubes then pour oil + herb mixture over top. Stir to coat.
4. Lay out on prepared cookie sheet and cook for 15-20 minutes (mine took 19 minutes) or until golden and slightly hard to the touch.
5. Remove from oven and let cool for 10-15 minutes. Store in the fridge in an airtight container for up to 5 days. *Serves 4*

Snap Pea and Quinoa Salad
2 cups water
1 cup quinoa
2 cups fresh snap peas, trimmed and cut diagonally into thirds
1 ½ cups button mushrooms, cut into quarters or eighths if large
1/3 cup thinly sliced red onion, cut into 1-inch lengths
1 T. chopped fresh dill
1/3 cup white balsamic vinegar or white-wine vinegar
¼ cup extra-virgin olive oil or flaxseed oil
1 tsp. freshly grated lemon zest
1 T. lemon juice
1 tsp. pure maple syrup

1. Combine water and quinoa in a medium saucepan. Bring to a boil.
2. Reduce to a simmer, cover and cook for 15 minutes.
3. Fluff with a fork and set aside to cool completely.
4. Combine peas, mushrooms, onion and dill in a medium bowl.

5. Whisk vinegar, oil, lemon zest, lemon juice and maple syrup in a small bowl.
6. Stir the dressing into the cooled quinoa until evenly dispersed.
7. Add the quinoa to the vegetable mixture, toss and serve. *Serves 6*

Mediterranean Lentil Salad

¾ cup dried green lentils (you want to end up with 2 cups cooked)
2 cups water
3 oz. canned/jar roasted red peppers, chopped
2 T. finely minced onion
2 medium cloves garlic, pressed
½ cup chopped fresh basil
1/3 cup coarsely chopped walnuts
3 T. balsamic vinegar
1 T. fresh lemon juice
2 T. + 2 T. extra virgin olive oil
Salt and pepper to taste
1 bunch arugula, chopped

1. Wash lentils, remove any foreign matter, and drain.
2. Combine lentils and 2 cups lightly salted water in medium saucepan. Bring to a boil.
3. Reduce heat, and cook at low temperature for about 20 minutes, or until lentils are cooked but still firm. Cook gently so lentils don't get mushy.
4. When done, drain any excess water, and lightly rinse under cold water. Continue to drain excess water.
5. Mince onion, press garlic and let sit for 5 minutes to bring out their hidden health-promoting benefits.
6. Place lentils in a bowl and add peppers, onion, garlic, basil, walnuts, vinegar, and
   2 T. olive oil. Season with salt and pepper to taste.
7. Marinate for at least 1 hour before serving.
8. Toss arugula with 2 T. olive oil, 1 T. lemon juice, salt and pepper.
9. Serve on plate with lentils. *Serves 4*

Asian Cabbage and Peanut Slaw
2 cups thinly sliced or shredded Napa cabbage
2 cups thinly sliced or shredded curly kale
2 cups shredded carrots
1 cup raw peanuts

Dressing:
¼ cup sesame oil
¼ cup lime or lemon juice
2 T. rice wine vinegar
1 T. Tamari soy sauce
½ T. honey

1. Combine veggies in a bowl.
2. Mix together dressing ingredients in a jar and shake well.
3. Pour dressing over veggies and toss well to combine.
4. Let sit for 20-30 minutes.
5. Mix in peanuts and serve. *Serves 4*

Wilted Kale Salad with a Creamy Chipotle Dressing
11 oz. kale
½ tsp. fine sea salt
1 cup baby tomatoes, sliced
½ cup hulled hemp seeds (hemp hearts)

Dressing:
2 avocados
1 jalapeno pepper*
¼ cup olive oil
2 T. lemon juice
Optional: a little warm water if needed to blend the dressing and make it creamy
*If not using the jalapeno pepper, substitute with ½ tsp. each of onion powder, cumin, chili powder, garlic powder and soy sauce.

1. Remove the stems and then wash and cut the kale into small pieces.

2. Place in a bowl, add salt and start to massage the kale until it wilts and takes on a 'cooked' texture.
3. Add the tomatoes and hemp seeds to the bowl and mix in by hand.
4. Blend all dressing ingredients in a blender until creamy and mix into kale by hand. *Serves 2*

Lemony Cabbage Avocado Slaw (RAW)

6 cups finely shredded purple and green cabbage
1 small red, orange or yellow pepper, chopped
1 ripe avocado, diced
2 T. red onion, finely chopped
3 T. lemon juice
¼ cup hulled hemp seeds
3 T. cilantro leaves
¼ tsp. sea salt

1. Toss all ingredients together in a large bowl until avocado is creamy throughout. *Serves 6*

Strawberry and Fava Bean Salad

Pinch of kosher or sea salt
2 cups shelled fresh fava beans (about 2 pounds in pods)
2 T. extra virgin olive oil
2 T. balsamic vinegar
2 T. lemon juice
2 cups fresh strawberries, stemmed and quartered
Coarsely ground black pepper
3 cups arugula
½ cup feta cheese

1. In a large pot over high heat, bring 2 quarts of water to a boil. Add a pinch of salt and the fava beans. Boil 1 minute; drain and cool fava beans in ice water. Drain fava beans;
2. pinch one end and slip off tough skins of larger beans (skin on small beans is not usually tough). Discard skins.
3. Whisk together olive oil, vinegar and lemon juice.

4. In a large bowl, season shelled fava beans and strawberries with salt and pepper.
5. Add arugula and enough dressing to coat salad lightly. Mix gently and spoon onto a platter or 6 salad plates. Sprinkle feta cheese generously over salad. Grind more pepper on top. *Serves 6*

LUNCH

Veggie Tacos
2 T. extra virgin olive oil
¾ lb. zucchini, trimmed and diced
3 scallions, trimmed and sliced
2 tsp. chili powder
¼ tsp. ground cumin
¼ tsp. dried oregano
¼ tsp. salt
¼ tsp. pepper
1 can kidney beans, drained and rinsed
1 can corn, drained and rinsed or just take the kernels off a few ears of fresh corn
2 cups baby spinach, chopped
¾ cup salsa
1 package of corn taco shells
⅔ cup feta cheese
Lime wedges

1. Heat oil in a large non-stick skillet over medium heat.
2. Add zucchini and scallions and cook 5 minutes.
3. Add chili powder, cumin, oregano, salt and pepper. Cook 1 minute.
4. Stir in beans, corn, spinach and salsa. Cook a few minutes until spinach wilts. Meanwhile, heat taco shells in foil in oven at 350°F (or in microwave per package instructions).
5. Spoon about ⅓ cup veggie mixture into each taco shell and sprinkle with cheese. Squeeze lime wedges over tacos and serve. *Makes 12 tacos*

Miso Avocado Open Faced Sandwich (FERMENTED)
1 avocado
1 heaping T. gluten free miso
Sprouts
Gluten free bread or rice cake of your choice

1. Remove skin from avocado and chop. Add to a small bowl with miso. *(cont.)*

2. Using a fork, mash together the miso and avocado.
3. Serve on toasted bread with sprouts. *Serves 1*

Pineapple Cucumber Gazpacho

4 cups pineapple, chopped
4 cups cucumber, peeled and chopped
3 T. jalapeno, minced
3 T. green onion, thinly sliced
1 T. lime juice
1 cup fresh pineapple juice
2 tsp. sea salt
½ cup loosely packed cilantro leaves
½ cup macadamia nuts, finely chopped
3 T. extra virgin olive oil

1. Add to a blender 3 cups each of the pineapple and cucumber, 2 T. of jalapeno, 2 T. green onion, lime juice, pineapple juice and salt and blend at high speed until smooth.
2. Taste for seasoning. Because the sweetness of pineapples varies, the amount of jalapeno and salt may need to be increased accordingly.
3. Add the remaining pineapple, cucumber, the cilantro leaves and 1½ T. of the olive oil. Pulse the blender quickly a few times - the gazpacho should remain chunky.
4. Add the macadamia nuts and stir to distribute them evenly.
5. Divide among serving bowls and drizzle with the olive oil and sprinkle with remaining minced jalapeno and sliced green onion. *Serves 4*

Black Bean Lettuce Cups

8 lettuce leaves (your favorite lettuce – except for iceberg; romaine, butter lettuce, etc.)
1 15 oz. can of black beans, drained and rinsed
½ cup fresh salsa (you can make it or buy it at the store)
Small handful of cilantro, chopped
1 avocado

Juice of one lime

Sea salt

1. Mash beans and salsa together in a bowl.
2. Add the chopped cilantro.
3. Spoon into lettuce cups.
4. Top with diced avocado and a squeeze of lime juice.
5. Season with salt. *Serves 2*

Romaine Lettuce Wraps

2 large Romaine leaves
1 shredded carrot
Handful of alfalfa sprouts
Red onion, sliced
Hummus or guacamole
Salt and pepper to taste

1. Wash and flatten the leaves.
2. Spread the center with hummus or guacamole.
3. Layer carrots, onions and sprouts.
4. Add salt and pepper.
5. Roll up the leaves to make a wrap. *Serves 2*

DINNER

Stuffed Autumn Squash

3 acorn squash
1 T. maple syrup
½ cup walnuts
2 tsp. canola oil
1 large onion, finely chopped
1 stalk of celery, thinly sliced
1 Granny Smith apple, cut into ¼-inch cubes
1/3 cup golden raisins, chopped
¼ cup uncooked quinoa (rinsed)
¾ cup chicken broth
¼ tsp. ground cinnamon
¼ tsp. salt

1. Heat oven to 400°F.
2. Place foil on a cookie sheet.
3. Cut the squash lengthwise, seed, then brush cut surfaces and inside with maple syrup. Arrange squash, cut-side down, on pan and bake in 400°F oven for 30-40 minutes, until tender.
4. Meanwhile, toast walnuts, chopped, in nonstick skillet over medium heat, stirring, 5 minutes or until golden and transfer to paper towel.
5. Heat canola oil in same skillet over medium-high heat; add the finely chopped large onion and the sliced celery.
6. Sauté 3 minutes, until just tender.
7. Add the Granny Smith apple, golden raisins, quinoa, chicken broth, ground cinnamon, and salt.
8. Cover; simmer 15 minutes, until quinoa is tender and liquid absorbed.
9. Stir in toasted walnuts and reduce oven to 350°F.
10. Flip squash cut-side up, fill with apple mixture, and drizzle with 1 tablespoon syrup.
11. Bake in 350°F oven for 15 minutes. *Serves 6*

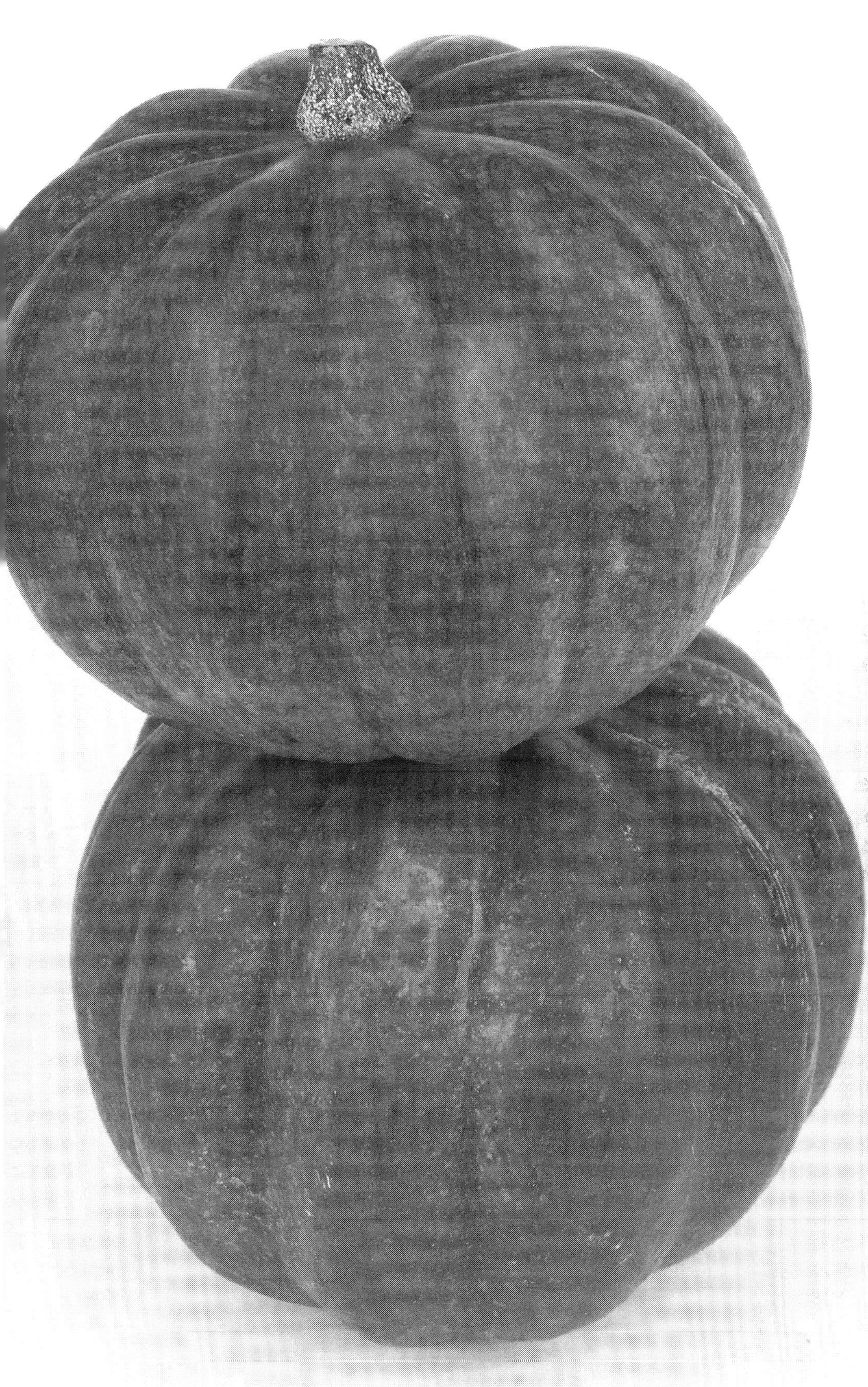

Chunky Vegetable-Lentil Soup
1 T. olive oil
1 medium onion, cut into thin rings
1 clove garlic, minced
1 cup dry green (French) lentils, rinsed and drained
1 lb. whole small mushrooms (halve or quarter any larger mushrooms)
4 medium carrots, thinly sliced (2 cups)
2 stalks celery, chopped
4 cups water
1 14-oz. can vegetable broth
¼ tsp. salt
¼ tsp. ground black pepper
¼ of a head Napa or red cabbage, sliced into strips (2 cups)

1. In a large saucepan, heat oil over medium heat.
2. Add onion and garlic, cook for 4-5 minutes until tender, stirring occasionally.
3. Add lentils and stir 1 minute.
4. Add mushrooms, carrots, celery, water, broth, salt and pepper. Bring to a boil.
5. Reduce heat and simmer, covered for 25 minutes or until lentils are tender.
6. Divide among bowls and top with cabbage. *Serves 6*

Bean and Vegetable Stew
1 large onion, diced
2 celery stalks, diced
2 cloves garlic, minced
1 T. canola oil
5 cups vegetable broth
1 tsp. sage
1 tsp. thyme
1 tsp. rosemary
2 bay leaves
¼ cup Tamari or Braggs
2 cups pumpkin or other squash, chopped in ½" cubes
2 cups carrots, coarsely chopped
2 cups green beans cut in 1" pieces
1 small head of cabbage or ½ large head, coarsely

chopped.
3 cups cooked beans (any variety), drained
¼ cup cornstarch mixed with ½ cup water

1. Sauté onion, celery and garlic in 1 T. oil for 4 minutes.
2. Add 5 cups of vegetable broth, sage, thyme, rosemary, bay leaves, soy sauce, pumpkin and carrots.
3. Bring to a boil and cook for 15 minutes.
4. Add green beans and cabbage, and cook until beans are tender.
5. Add 3 cups of other beans and cornstarch mixture, stirring constantly.
6. Bring to a boil.
7. Prepare the dumplings (if using – see next page) and drop by tablespoon into hot stew (about 8 dumplings). Cover and cook for 12 minutes or until dumplings are done. Do not lift the lid during this final cooking time.
8. Remove bay leaves and serve immediately.

Portobello Curry with Green Rice

1 cup basmati rice
1 cup unsweetened coconut milk
½ cup snipped fresh cilantro
4 tsp. finely minced fresh ginger
2 cloves garlic, minced
1 T. lime juice
1 lb. Portobello mushrooms, cut in ½-inch slices
2 T. vegetable oil
½ cup sliced green onions
2 tsp. curry powder
1/8 tsp. crushed red pepper
1 cup cherry tomatoes, halved or quartered
2 T. coarsely chopped cashews or peanuts

1. In medium saucepan, combine rice, 2 cups water, and ½ teaspoon salt. Bring to boil and then reduce heat.
2. Simmer, covered, 15 to 20 minutes or until rice is tender and liquid is absorbed.
3. Meanwhile, in blender or food processor combine ½ cup of the coconut milk, the cilantro, 1 tsp. of *(cont.)*

the ginger, 1 garlic clove, and the lime juice. Cover; blend or process until nearly smooth.
4. Stir into rice.
5. Cover; keep warm.
6. In 12-inch skillet, cook mushrooms in hot oil over medium heat for 5 minutes; turn occasionally. Add green onions, curry powder, red pepper, and remaining ginger and garlic. Cook and stir 1 minute.
7. Stir in tomatoes and remaining coconut milk.
8. Heat through.
9. Season to taste with salt and black pepper.
10. To serve, divide rice among plates. Top with mushroom mixture and sprinkle with nuts. *Serves 4*

Italian Tofu Frittata

Frittatas are great for a dinner but save some leftovers for breakfast or lunch.

1 cup onion, chopped fine
4 cloves garlic, minced
1 cup zucchini, diced
1 cup red bell pepper, diced
2 cups finely chopped kale (remove stems)
1 cup fresh tomato
¼ cup plus 2 T. chicken or vegetable broth
2 T. red wine vinegar
5 oz. firm tofu, drained
4 egg whites
1 T. dried Italian seasoning (I like Emeril's)
¼ tsp. turmeric
Salt and pepper to taste
2 T. chopped fresh parsley

1. Chop all vegetables.
2. Puree tofu with egg whites, Italian seasoning and turmeric in blender.
3. In a 10" stainless steel pan, heat 2 T. broth.
4. When broth begins to steam, add onion, garlic, zucchini, pepper, kale and tomato.
5. Sauté for about 1 minute over medium heat, stirring often.

6. Add ¼ cup broth and red wine vinegar.
7. Pour tofu mixture over vegetables and cover.
8. Cook over low heat until mixture is completely firm and cooked, about 12 minutes.
9. Top with chopped parsley and salt and pepper to taste.
10. Serve with Baked Parmesan Tomatoes and salad of your choice. *Serves 4*

Quick Broiled Chicken

2 6-oz boneless chicken breasts (skin on)
2 tsp. fresh lemon juice
Sea salt and pepper to taste

Dressing:
2 cloves garlic, chopped
3 T. extra virgin olive oil
2 tsp. fresh lemon juice
Sea salt and pepper to taste
Optional: Add rosemary, sage or Dijon mustard to dressing and/or top with sautéed mushrooms

1. Preheat the broiler on high and place an all stainless steel skillet or cast iron pan about 6 inches from the heat for about 10 minutes to get it very hot.
2. While the pan is heating, rinse and pat the chicken dry and season with lemon juice, salt, and pepper.
3. Leaving the skin on, place the breast skin side up on the hot pan and return it to the oven. (It is not necessary to turn the breast because it is cooking on both sides at once. Depending on the size, it should be cooked in about 7 minutes.
4. Remove the skin before serving; it is left on to keep it moist while broiling. The breast is done when it is moist, yet its liquid runs clear when pierced. The inside temperature needs to reach 165°F.
5. Dress with garlic, lemon juice, extra virgin olive oil, salt, and pepper. Add rosemary, sage, or Dijon mustard to the dressing if desired. You can also top with sautéed mushrooms for extra flavor. *Serves 2*

Lemon Tofu
2 T. olive oil, divided
2 x 8 oz. packages cubed super firm tofu, drained
Grated zest of 2 lemons
3 cloves garlic
½ tsp. crushed red pepper flakes, or to taste
1 medium red onion, halved and thinly sliced
2 medium bell peppers, thinly sliced
2 T. mirin (rice wine) or water
1 cup coconut milk
1 T. gluten free soy sauce
1 tsp. honey
¼ tsp. salt, or to taste
1 x 12 oz. pkg. fresh or frozen trimmed green beans
1 cup basil or cilantro leaves, shredded
1 lime, cut into wedges (optional garnish)

1. Heat 1 T. of the oil over medium-high heat in a large nonstick skillet until very hot.
2. Fry tofu until golden, about 3 to 5 minutes. Turn over and fry on other side. Remove tofu and drain on a paper towel-lined plate.
3. Mix lemon zest, garlic and red pepper flakes. Add remaining 1 T. oil to skillet and heat over medium heat.
4. Add lemon zest mixture, onion and bell peppers. Cook over medium-low heat, stirring, for about 1 minute, until fragrant.
5. Add mirin, wine, or water, stir, and partially cover. Cook until onions are tender, about 5 minutes.
6. Add coconut milk, soy sauce, honey, and salt and stir to mix. Cover and bring to a boil over high heat.
7. Reduce heat to maintain a simmer, add green beans, and stir.
8. If desired, thin the stew with a few tablespoons of water. Cover and cook until beans are tender, about 6 minutes.
9. Uncover and add reserved tofu and basil or cilantro. Heat over medium heat until tofu is warmed through.
10. Transfer to a serving bowl and serve hot, garnished with lime wedges if desired. *Serves 4*

Poached Eggs Over Collard Greens & Shiitake Mushrooms

6 cups chopped collard greens (stems removed)
1 medium onion, cut in half and sliced thin
6 fresh shiitake mushrooms, sliced medium thick, stems removed
4 eggs
About 4 cups water
1 T. apple cider vinegar or any white wine vinegar

Dressing:
1 T. fresh lemon juice
1 T. minced fresh ginger
3 medium cloves garlic pressed
1 T. soy sauce
1 T. extra virgin olive oil
Salt and white pepper to taste

1. Slice onions and press garlic.
2. Bring lightly salted water to a boil in a steamer.
3. Rinse greens well. Roll or stack leaves and cut into ½ inch slices and cut again crosswise. Cut stem into ¼ inch slices.
4. Steam collard greens, mushrooms and onions together for 5 minutes. While steaming greens, get ready for poaching eggs by bringing water and vinegar to a fast simmer in a small, shallow pan.
5. You can start on high heat, and once it comes to a boil, reduce heat to a simmer before adding eggs. Make sure there is enough water to cover eggs.
6. Mix together lemon juice, ginger, garlic, soy sauce, olive oil, salt, and pepper in a small bowl.
7. Poach eggs until desired doneness. This will take about 5 minutes, or just until the white is set and the yolk has filmed over.
8. Remove vegetables from steamer and toss with dressing.
9. Remove eggs from water with a slotted spoon and place on plate of tossed greens. *Serves 4*

Asian Meatball Soup with Kale and Rice Noodles

Note: Adding the kale toward the end of cooking preserves its bright green color, as well as its nutrients. Chopping kale releases its antioxidants.

4 cups chicken broth
4 quarter-size slices fresh ginger
1 tsp. grated fresh ginger
12 oz. lean ground turkey or chicken
1 egg white
2 T. plain gluten free dry bread crumbs
1½ tsp. minced garlic
2½ tsp. soy sauce
3 cups trimmed, chopped, firmly packed kale leaves
1 x 8 oz. pkg. thin rice noodles
1½ tsp. toasted sesame oil
2 scallions, thinly sliced (optional)

1. In a large saucepan, combine broth and ginger slices. Bring to a simmer over medium-high heat.
2. In a separate saucepan, bring 3 quarts water to a boil over high heat for cooking the rice noodles. While broth heats, make meatballs.
3. In a large bowl, mix together grated ginger, ground turkey, egg white, bread crumbs, garlic, and soy sauce. Form into 16 to 20 meatballs (a small ice cream scoop works well for this).
4. Remove ginger slices from broth with a slotted spoon and discard.
5. Place meatballs in the broth, being careful not to crowd them. Bring to a gentle boil over medium-high heat.
6. Reduce heat to medium-low, cover, and simmer gently for 10 minutes.
7. Add kale. Cover and simmer 10 more minutes, until meatballs are cooked through and kale is tender.
8. After adding kale to the broth, drop rice noodles into pot with boiling water. Cook for 3 minutes. Drain, and then divide noodles among 4 bowls.
9. Stir sesame oil and scallions into broth.
10. Divide broth and meatballs among the 4 bowls. Serve at once. *Serves 4*

Stir-Fried Seafood with Asparagus
1 medium onion, cut in half and sliced medium thick
1 T. chicken or vegetable broth
1 T. minced fresh ginger
3 medium cloves garlic, chopped
2 cups fresh sliced shiitake mushrooms
1 bunch thin asparagus, cut in 2 inch lengths (discard bottom ¼)
¼ cup fresh lemon juice
2 T. Tamari (soy sauce)
2 T. mirin wine
Pinch red pepper flakes
¾ lb. cod fillet cut into 1 inch pieces
8 large scallops
8 large shrimp, peeled and deveined
1 cup cherry tomatoes cut in quarters
¼ cup chopped fresh cilantro
Salt and white pepper to taste

1. Slice onion and chop garlic.
2. Heat 1 T. broth in a stainless steel wok or 12 inch skillet.
3. Stir-fry onion in broth over medium high heat for 2 minutes, stirring constantly.
4. Add ginger, garlic, mushrooms and asparagus.

Continue to stir-fry for another 3 minutes, stirring constantly.

5. Add lemon juice, Tamari, mirin, red pepper flakes, cod, scallops, and shrimp and stir to mix well.
6. Cover and simmer for just about 5 minutes, stirring occasionally on medium heat.
7. Toss in tomatoes, cilantro, salt and pepper. Serve.

Serves 4

Spaghetti Squash Primavera
1 spaghetti squash (about 1½ lb.)
2 cloves garlic, peeled and minced
1 small onion, finely chopped
1 small zucchini, diced
2 tsp. extra virgin olive oil
1 can (28 oz.) diced plum tomatoes (Muir Glen Organic is my favorite)

(cont.)

1 tsp. apple cider vinegar
1 tsp. dried oregano
1 tsp. dried basil
½ tsp. red pepper flakes
Fresh basil

1. Preheat oven to 375°F.
2. Halve squash lengthwise and scoop out seeds.
3. Cover a sided baking sheet or Pyrex dish with foil. Lay halves, flesh side down, on sheet. Add about ¼ inch of water. Cover with foil.
4. Bake 35 minutes or until you can easily pierce shell.
5. While squash bakes, sauté garlic, onion, and zucchini in oil over medium heat 5 minutes. Add remaining ingredients except fresh basil and cook, stirring occasionally, for 30 minutes. Lower heat if sauce begins to boil.
6. Remove squash from oven. Scrape crosswise to pull strands from shell.
7. Place squash in 4 serving bowls. Pour sauce over squash and garnish with basil. *Serves 4*

Zesty Mexican Soup
1 medium onion, minced
4 medium cloves garlic, chopped
2 T. red chili powder
3 cups + 1 T. chicken or vegetable broth
1 small to medium green bell pepper, diced into ¼ inch pieces
1 small zucchini, diced into ¼ inch pieces
1 cup collard greens, finely chopped
1 15 oz. can diced tomatoes
1 15 oz. can black beans, rinsed
1 cup frozen yellow corn
1 4 oz. can diced green chili
1 tsp. dried oregano
1 tsp. ground cumin
¼ cup pumpkin seeds, chopped
½ cup fresh cilantro, chopped
Salt and pepper to taste
Optional: Dollop of non-dairy sour cream (i.e. cashew sour cream)

1. Heat 1T. broth in a medium soup pot. Sauté onion, garlic and green peppers in broth over medium heat for about 5 minutes, stirring often.
2. Add red chili powder and mix in well. Add broth, zucchini, collard greens, and tomatoes.
3. Cook for another 5 minutes and add beans, corn, green chili, oregano, and cumin. Bring to a boil on high heat. Once it begins to boil, reduce heat to medium-low and simmer uncovered for 15 minutes longer. (Simmering uncovered enhances the flavor.) Add chopped cilantro, pumpkin seeds, salt, and pepper. *Serves 6*

Black Bean Burgers

2 ½ cups of cooked black beans
1 cup gluten free bread crumbs
4 eggs
½ tsp. sea salt
½ tsp. cumin
½ tsp. chili powder
¼ tsp. oregano
¼ tsp. dried cilantro or 2 T. chopped fresh cilantro
½ small chopped onion or 1 tsp. onion powder
1 tsp. garlic powder

1. In a food processor combine all ingredients and puree until the mixture is well combined.
2. Form into burgers (whatever size you prefer) and pan fry in a covered, oiled heavy skillet for 5-10 minutes per side depending on your burger size.

Note: These can be served on gluten free buns but my favorite way to eat them (since there is already bread in the burger) is plated with peach salsa and a sprout or garden salad.

Peach Salsa:
4 large peaches diced, pitted and skin removed
½ a red onion, diced
1-2 jalapenos, diced
½ bunch cilantro, chopped
Juice of 1 large lime *(cont.)*

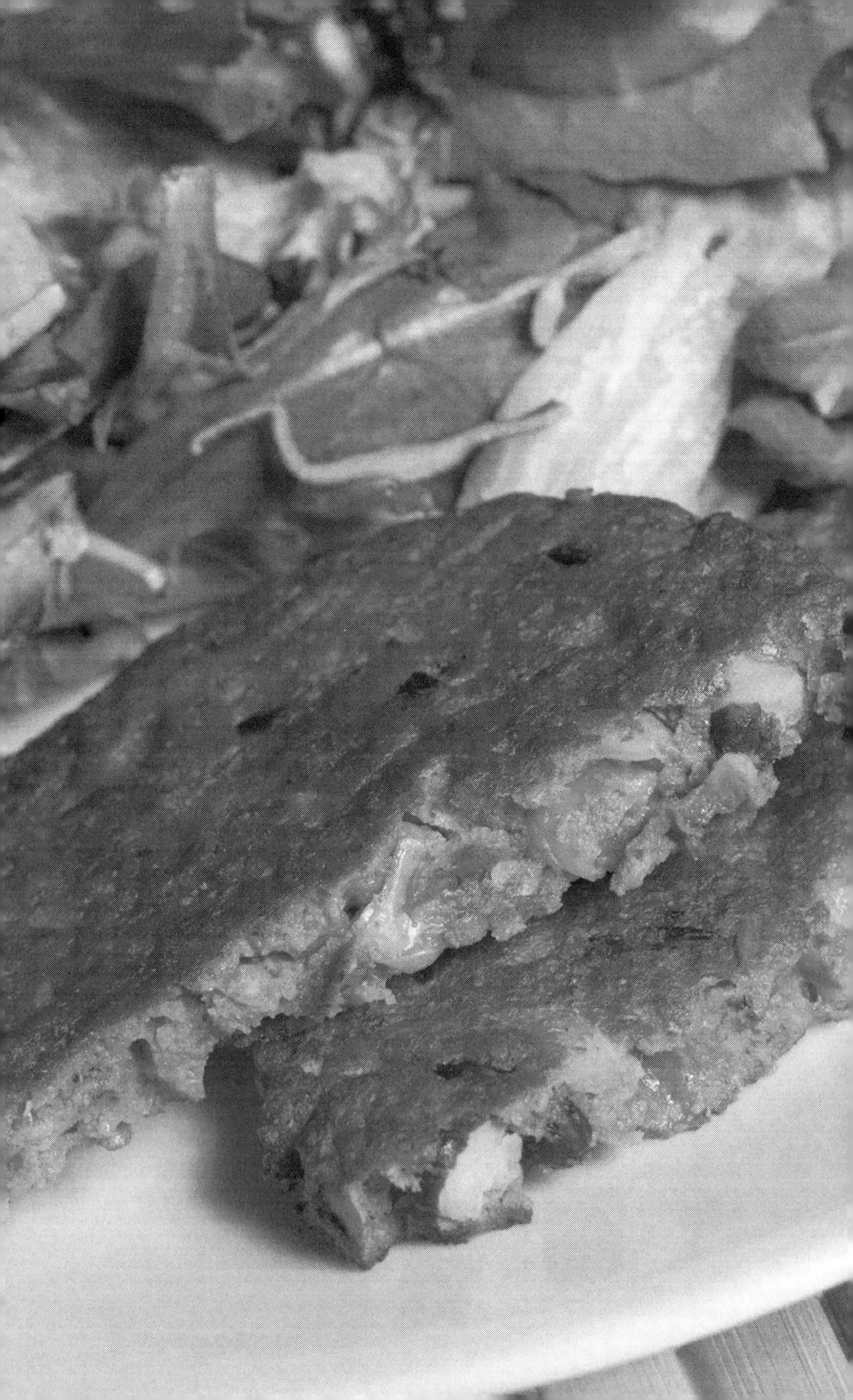

Salt and pepper to taste

1. In a large bowl, add the peaches, red onion, jalapeno, cilantro, and fresh lime juice. Stir well.
2. Season with salt and pepper.
3. Serve over the burgers or with chicken, fish, or any Mexican dish. *Serves 4*

Miso Salmon (FERMENTED)
1 lb. salmon, cut into 4 pieces, skin and bones removed
2 tsp. gluten free miso
1 T. prepared Dijon mustard
2 T. mirin (Japanese rice cooking wine found in Asian section of market)
4 dried medium size pieces of wakame seaweed, rinsed and soaked in ½ cup hot water for about 10 minutes (save the soaking water)
1 medium onion, cut in half and sliced
3 cups sliced fresh shiitake mushrooms
3 medium cloves garlic, chopped
½ T. minced fresh ginger
2 tsp. Tamari (soy sauce)
Salt and white pepper to taste
Minced green onion (for garnish)

1. Rinse and soak seaweed, saving the water.
2. Slice onion and chop garlic.
3. Prepare glaze by mixing miso, Dijon mustard, and mirin along with a pinch of white pepper.
4. Generously coat salmon with mixture and let set while preparing rest of ingredients.
5. Heat 1 T. seaweed water in a stainless steel skillet.
6. Sauté onion, garlic, ginger, and mushrooms in broth over medium heat for about 5 minutes.
7. Add chopped seaweed, ½ cup seaweed water and Tamari and cook for another 5 minutes. Season with salt and pepper.
8. Broil without turning for about 3-5 minutes depending on thickness of salmon.
9. Top with sautéed onion/mushroom mixture and minced scallion. *Serves 4*

Raw Pad Thai (RAW and FERMENTED)
2 zucchini, ends trimmed
2 carrots, sliced in to long strips
1 head red cabbage, thinly sliced
1 red bell pepper, thinly sliced
½ cup bean sprouts
¾ cup raw almond butter
2 oranges, juiced
2 T. raw honey
1 T. minced fresh ginger root
1 T. soy sauce
1 T. gluten free miso
1 clove garlic, minced
¼ tsp. cayenne pepper

1. Slice zucchini lengthwise with a vegetable peeler to create long thin 'noodles'. Place on individual plates.
2. Slice carrots into long strips with vegetable peeler similar to the zucchini.
3. Combine carrots, cabbage, red bell pepper, and bean sprouts in a large bowl.
4. Whisk together almond butter, orange juice, honey, ginger, soy sauce, miso, garlic, and cayenne pepper in a bowl. Pour half of sauce into cabbage mixture and toss to coat.
5. Top zucchini 'noodles' with cabbage mixture.
6. Pour remaining sauce over each portion. *Serves 4*

Primavera Verde
The vegetables you use are only limited by your imagination and it's a great way to use whatever is in your refrigerator. Enjoy!

1 medium onion, quartered and sliced thin
1 small red bell pepper, cut in 1 inch strips
1 medium carrot, cut in very thin sticks 1 ½ inches long
1 bunch thin asparagus, cut 1 ½ inches long, discard bottom fourth
1 ½ cups zucchini or summer yellow squash, cut in thin 1 inch strips

6 medium cloves garlic, chopped
1 x 15 oz. can diced tomatoes, with juice
1 T. + ¼ cup vegetable broth
1 cup fresh basil, chopped
3 T. fresh sage, minced
1 cup fresh parsley, minced
3 T. fresh oregano, minced
Salt and black pepper to taste
4 oz. gluten free pasta of your choice
Optional: 4 oz. Chevre goat cheese

1. Bring salted water to a boil for pasta.
2. Chop all vegetables as listed.
3. Heat 1 T. broth in skillet. Sauté onion in broth over medium heat, stirring frequently for 3 minutes.
4. Add fresh vegetables in order given, waiting about 1 minute between each.
5. Add tomatoes and broth and simmer for another couple of minutes, until vegetables are barely tender, about 10 minutes. If needed, you can add a touch more liquid to keep moist.
6. Add minced herbs.
7. Season with salt and pepper.
8. While vegetables are simmering, cook pasta according to package instructions and strain through colander.
9. Toss pasta with vegetable mixture and top with goat cheese if desired. *Serves 6*

Brown Rice and Goat Cheese Cakes

¾ cup brown rice
1½ cups water
4 tsp. extra virgin olive oil, divided
6 medium shallots, chopped
2 medium carrots, shredded using the large holes of a box grater
½ cup pecans, toasted
3 oz. goat cheese
1 large egg white
½ tsp. dried thyme
½ tsp. salt
½ tsp. ground black pepper *(cont.)*

1. Bring rice and water to a boil in a medium saucepan. Reduce heat to low, cover, and simmer until the water is absorbed and the rice is tender, 30 to 50 minutes.
2. Remove from the heat and let stand, covered, for 10 minutes.
3. Meanwhile, heat 2 tsp. oil in a large skillet over medium heat.
4. Add shallots; cook, stirring often, until soft, 2 to 3 minutes.
5. Add carrots, reduce the heat to low and cook, stirring often, until softened and the shallots are lightly browned, about 4 minutes. Remove from the heat.
6. Preheat oven to 400°F. Transfer the cooked vegetables and rice to a large food processor.
7. Add pecans, goat cheese, egg white, thyme, salt and pepper. Pulse until well blended but still a little coarse. Scrape into a large bowl.
8. With wet hands, form the mixture into six 3-inch patties (about ½ cup each).
9. Heat the remaining 2 tsp. oil in a large nonstick skillet over medium heat.
10. Add the patties and cook until well browned, 3 to 4 minutes per side.
11. Transfer to a baking sheet and bake 10 to 15 minutes. *Makes 6 cakes*

Slow Cooker Green Chicken Chili with Kale

2 cups dried great northern beans, soaked for 24 hours in plenty of water
1 large onion, chopped
5 garlic cloves, minced
8 cups chicken stock
1 T. cumin
1/8 – 1/4 tsp. cayenne, depending on your taste
2 (4.5 oz.) cans green chilies, chopped
2 cups cooked, cubed chicken
1 bunch of kale, leaves stripped from the stalks and chopped
Sea salt to taste

Garnish: Dollop of goat yogurt, scallions, cilantro

1. Drain and rinse the soaked beans.
2. Place beans in slow cooker (at least 4 ½ quart size).
3. Add onions, garlic, a good pinch of salt, cumin, cayenne and chicken stock to beans.
4. Simmer the beans with this mixture in the slow cooker for 5 hours, or until tender.
5. Mix in the green chilies and chicken and simmer for another 2 hours.
6. Thirty minutes before serving, stir in the chopped kale.
7. Taste for seasoning and adjust flavors with sea salt if needed (this will depend on whether or not your stock was salted).
8. Garnishes can include dollops of goat yogurt, sliced scallions and cilantro. *Serves 4*

Asian Stuffed Cabbage Rolls

1 lb. lean ground turkey
2 carrots, shredded
1 cup cooked brown rice
4-5 garlic cloves, finely minced
2 T. ginger, finely minced
1 small onion, minced
3 T. Tamari (gluten free soy sauce)
2 T. toasted sesame oil
1 – 2 splashes rice vinegar
1 tsp. chili sauce or pinch red pepper flakes, optional
Salt and pepper to taste
Leaves from 1 head of Napa cabbage

1. Preheat your oven to 400°F.
2. In a large mixing bowl, prepare your filling by combing the turkey, carrots, rice, garlic, ginger, onion, tamari, sesame oil, chili sauce or red pepper flakes (optional) and a pinch of salt and black pepper.
3. Take the leaves from your cabbage and roll with a rolling pin to make leaves more pliable.
4. Lay out one cabbage leaf at a time and fill with meat mixture. Roll up. *(cont.)*

5. Place cabbage bundles in a baking dish. Pour 1 cup of water over cabbage and cover with aluminum foil. Bake in your preheated oven for about 30-35 minutes or until completely cooked through. Serve with juices from baking dish and additional chili sauce. *Serves 4-6*

Time saving tip: Prepare rolls ahead of time (without water) and refrigerate until ready for baking.

Grilled Black Bean Burgers

2 cups cooked black beans (about 2 15-ounce cans), drained & rinsed
1¼ tsp. garlic powder
1 tsp. chili powder
1 tsp. cumin
½ tsp. ground paprika
½ tsp. salt
2 tsp. finely chopped cilantro
Pinch of turmeric (optional)
¼ cup green peppers, finely chopped
½ cup gluten free bread crumbs or oats
½ cup red onion, finely chopped
1 large carrot, grated
1 egg or 1 flax egg (see over)

1. In a large mixing bowl, mash 1½ cups of the black beans. Add remaining ½ cup of beans.
2. In a small bowl, mix together the garlic powder, chili powder, cumin, paprika, salt, cilantro, and turmeric (if using).
3. Pour the spices over the bean mixture.
4. Add all of the remaining ingredients, and mix well with your hands.
5. Form into four or five large patties.
6. Grill on a greased sheet of aluminum foil on the grill just as you would a traditional burger. (Use the foil to prevent pieces from falling down between the grates until it cooks thoroughly.) Or you can cook these burgers in a pan.
7. Once browned and starting to crisp on the bottom side,

flip and do the same on the other.

8. Serve on your favorite gluten free bun with toppings or over a bed of lettuce or over rice. *Serves 4*

How to make a flax egg:
1 T. ground flax + 3 T. warm water.
Mix and set aside for at least 5 minutes.

Green Curry and Coconut Soba Noodles
1 (8 oz.) package soba noodles (be sure to purchase a wheat-free variety)
2/3 cup almond butter
3 T. green curry paste (found in health food store)
1 cup coconut milk
1 T. Tamari (gluten free soy sauce)
¼ cup fresh mint or basil, chopped
¼ cup toasted pepitas (pumpkin seeds)

1. Boil soba noodles in a large saucepot. Drain noodles in a colander then return the pot to the warm burner.
2. Whisk together the almond butter, green curry paste, coconut milk, and Tamari in the warm pot until combined, then add the noodles back into the pot and stir to combine.
3. Transfer to a serving bowl and top with chopped mint and pepitas.
4. Serve and enjoy. Serves 2

Shrimp Tacos with Citrus Slaw
¼ small green cabbage, thinly sliced
1 red bell pepper, thinly sliced
½ small white onion, thinly sliced
¼ cup fresh lime juice (from 2-3 limes)
Salt and pepper
2 T. plus 1 tsp. extra virgin olive oil
1 ½ lbs. large shrimp, deveined, peeled and tails removed
½ tsp. ground chili powder
8 small gluten free tortillas, warmed

(cont.)

1. In a large bowl, combine the cabbage, pepper, onion, lime juice, 2 T. oil, and some salt and pepper. Let sit for at least 5 minutes, tossing occasionally.
2. Heat remaining tsp. oil in a large skillet over high heat.
3. Season shrimp with the chili powder and salt; cook until opaque throughout, about 2-3 minutes per side.
4. Fill the tortillas with the shrimp and the slaw. *Serves 4*

Avocado Pesto Pasta

1 lb. gluten free pasta
1 bunch fresh basil, reserving a few sprigs for garnish
½ cup pine nuts
2 avocados, peeled and pitted
2 T. fresh lemon juice
3 cloves garlic
½ cup olive oil
Salt and pepper
1 cup cherry tomatoes, halved

1. Bring a large pot of salted water to a boil.
2. Add pasta and cook according to package directions. Drain and set aside.
3. Combine basil, pine nuts, avocados, lemon juice, garlic, and oil in a food processor. Process until smooth. Season generously with salt and pepper.
4. Toss pasta with pesto; add tomatoes. Divide pasta among serving bowls and garnish each serving with a basil leaf. *Serves 4*

Pan-Seared Cod and Roasted Asparagus in Coconut Milk Broth

This might seem like a lot of steps and a lot of ingredients but this is one of my favorite fish dishes - so delicious!

For the asparagus
1 pound asparagus
1 T. olive oil
Salt and pepper to taste

1. Preheat the oven to 400°F.
2. Rinse the asparagus well. Break off the woody end of

each spear and discard.

3. On a rimmed baking sheet, toss the asparagus with the olive oil. Add salt and pepper to taste. Roast for 20 – 25 minutes, shaking pan halfway through, or until asparagus has browned on the edges and is tender.

For the coconut milk broth

2 T. coconut oil
3 shallots, peeled and minced
2 cloves garlic, peeled and minced
1 T. minced ginger
1 tsp. red chili paste
2 T. prepared green curry paste (found in the Asian section of grocery store)
2 cups chicken stock
14 oz. can full-fat coconut milk
Sea salt and black pepper to taste

1. Heat a large, wide sauté pan over medium-high heat. Add the coconut oil and then the shallots. Sauté for 4 minutes.
2. Add garlic, ginger, chili paste and curry paste, and cook for 2 minutes.
3. Pour in ¼ cup chicken stock and scrape up any brown bits. Pour in the remaining stock and coconut milk. Bring to a rolling boil, and then turn heat to low. Add salt and pepper to taste. Simmer for 20 minutes.

For the pan-seared cod

2 cod fillets, ½ inch thick
2 T. olive oil, divided
Salt and pepper to taste
Lime, minced cilantro or parsley, and scallions to taste

1. Rinse the cod and blot with paper towels. Sprinkle both sides of the cod with salt/ pepper.
2. Heat a medium sauté pan over medium-high heat. Add 1 T. olive oil. Sear the fish, cooking each side for 4 – 5 minutes, or until fish is cooked through. Add the remaining tablespoon of olive oil if needed.

(cont.)

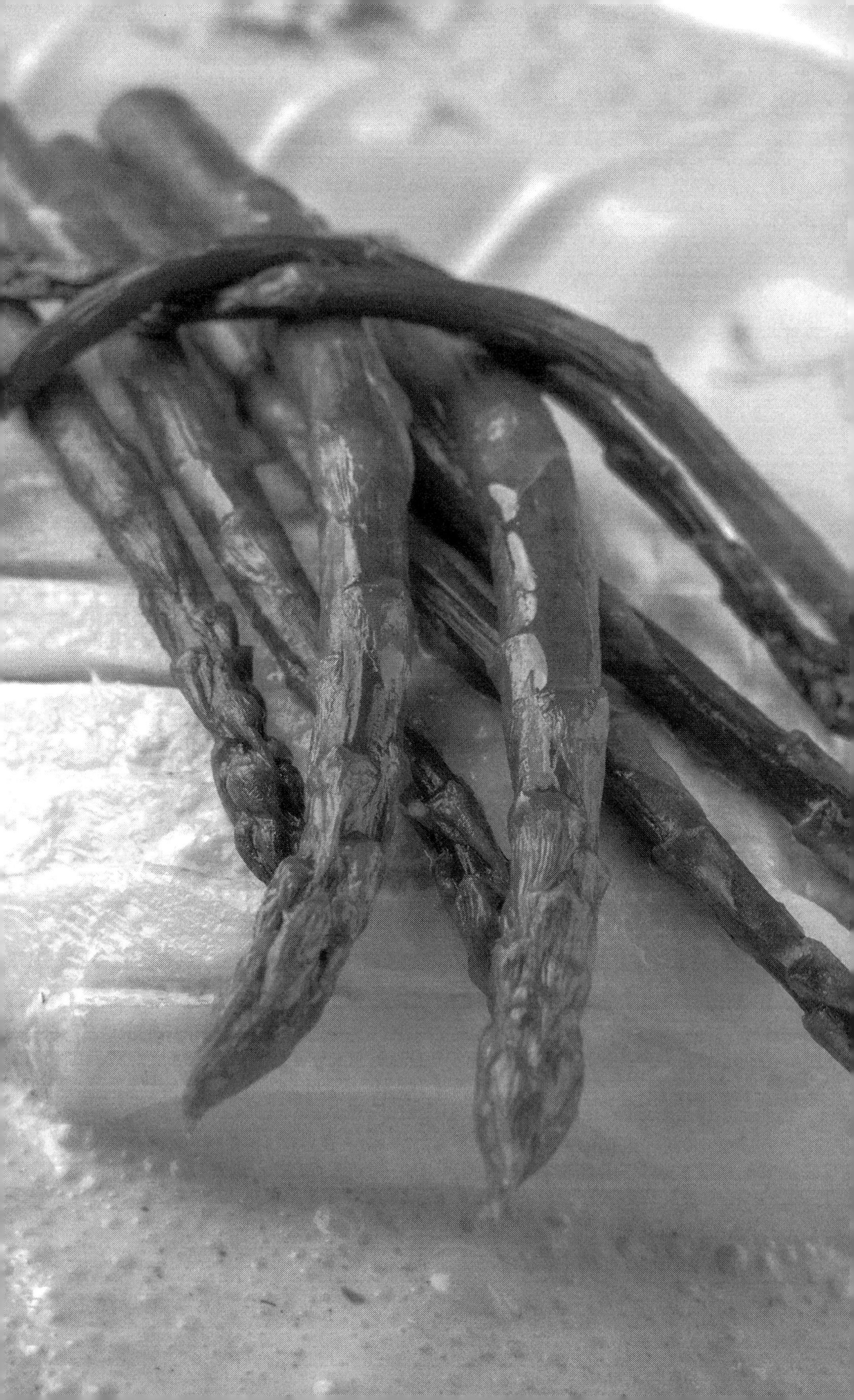

3. To serve, divide the asparagus between four shallow bowls. Top with cod and ladle the coconut broth over the dish.
4. Top dish off with a squeeze of lime, minced cilantro or parsley, and scallions. *Serves 2*

Orange Chicken Soba Noodles
2/3 cup orange juice
1/3 cup honey
1/3 cup soy sauce
1 tsp. garlic powder
½ tsp. ginger
½ lb. chicken, diced
1 sweet potato, cooked until tender then diced
1 zucchini or yellow squash, diced
2 eggs
½ (13.75 package) soba noodles, cooked (be sure that the soba noodles you purchase do not have wheat an added ingredient)
Fresh basil, chopped

1. In a wok (or deep frying pan), heat orange juice, honey, soy sauce, garlic powder, and ginger over high heat. Once boiling, toss in chicken, sweet potato, and zucchini. Cook until chicken is cooked through. Toss in soba noodles.
2. In a small skillet, scramble and cook eggs. Toss scrambled eggs into the soba noodle mixture.
3. Garnish with fresh basil, if desired. Serve and enjoy *Serves 4*

Vegan Mac and Cheese
2 ½ cups gluten free elbow macaroni
¼ cup non-dairy spread (such as Earth Balance)
¼ cup gluten free all-purpose flour
2 cups non-dairy milk
2 ½ cups shredded vegan cheese (I'm a fan of Daiya brand)
2 T. nutritional yeast*
Salt and pepper to taste

(cont.)

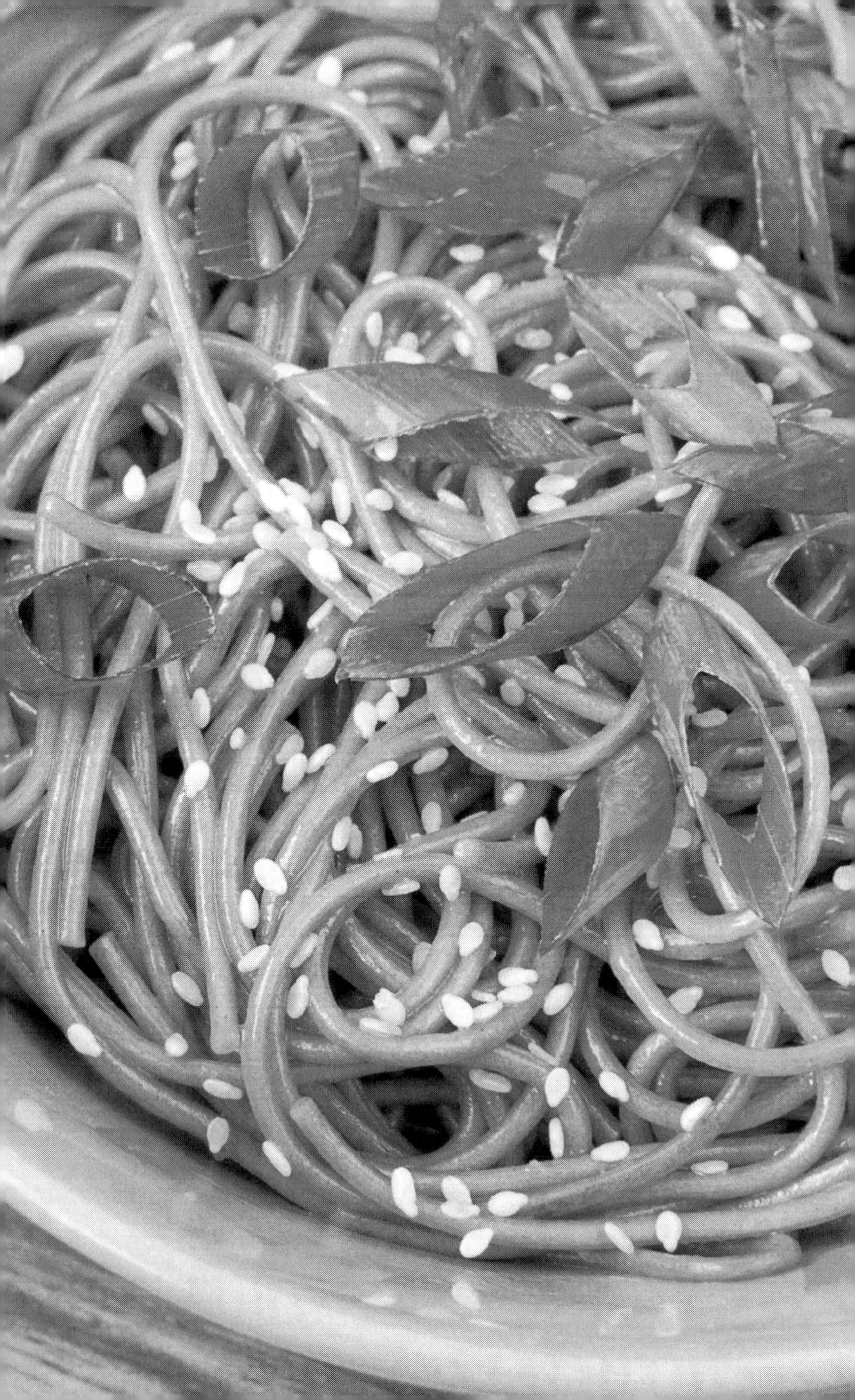

1 cup gluten free bread crumbs
1 T. oil

1. Pre-heat oven to 375 °F. Lightly grease a 2-quart oven -safe casserole dish.
2. Cook macaroni 1-2 minutes less than the package directions and drain.
3. Melt spread in a large skillet over medium heat. Whisk in flour and cook, continuing to whisk, until mixture is tan in color (about 3 minutes). Add milk slowly, whisking continuously, and bring to a boil. Boil for 1-2 minutes and gradually add 1 ½ cups of the shredded vegan cheese. Add 1 T. of the nutritional yeast, and salt and pepper to taste.
4. Add drained pasta and stir well to combine. Transfer to your prepared casserole dish.
5. In a small bowl combine the remaining 1 cup shredded cheese, 1 T. nutritional yeast, bread crumbs and salt and pepper to taste. Drizzle oil over and stir well to combine. Sprinkle topping over the pasta mixture.
6. Bake 30-40 minutes or until golden brown. Remove from oven and let sit for 10 minutes prior to serving.
   Serves: 4-6

**Wondering what nutritional yeast is? Long a staple in vegan cooking, it is an inactive yeast obtained from molasses, typically sold as flakes, that lends a taste and mouthfeel strikingly similar to Parmesan cheese. Most commonly found brands are Red Star and Bob's Red Mill.*

Asparagus. Pea and Leek Stir Fry
½ pound of asparagus, trimmed and sliced into 1 ½ inch pieces
½ pound sugar snap peas, trimmed
5 oz. frozen petite peas
¼ cup water
1 T. hoisin sauce
1 T .soy sauce
1 T. rice vinegar
1 tsp. sesame oil
½ tsp. cornstarch or arrowroot *(cont.)*

2 T. vegetable oil
1 leek, white part only, thinly sliced
1 T. minced ginger

1. Bring a large pot of water to a boil and boil the asparagus and sugar snap peas two minutes, adding the frozen peas for the last 10 seconds. Drain the vegetables into a strainer.
2. Combine the water, hoisin sauce, soy sauce, vinegar, sesame oil and the cornstarch. Stir to combine, making sure the cornstarch dissolves.
3. Heat a wok on high heat and add 1 T. of the vegetable oil. When the oil is heated, add the leek and ginger and stir for about two minutes.
4. Add the rest of the oil and stir in the vegetables and stir for about two minutes.
5. Add the sauce and stir for about one minute, until the sauce thickens.

Enjoy with steamed brown rice. *Serves 4.*

Loaded Baked Sweet Potatoes with Ginger Citrus Vinaigrette

4 6-inch garnet sweet potatoes (also called garnet yams)

1. Preheat the oven to 400°F. Wash the potatoes well, dry, and then poke all over with a fork. Wrap tightly with aluminum foil.
2. Set on a rimmed baking sheet and slide into the oven.
3. Bake for 50 – 60 minutes, or until sweet potatoes are fork tender.

Ginger Citrus Vinaigrette
3 T. extra virgin olive oil
2 T. apple cider vinegar
2 T. minced red onion
1 T. lime juice
1 T. lime zest
1 T. cilantro, minced
1 tsp. fresh ginger, minced
¼ tsp. sea salt
¼ tsp. ground cayenne (optional)

1. One at a time, whisk the ingredients into the olive oil. Set aside.

Toppings
Sea salt and pepper to taste
2 tangelos (or clementines, navel oranges, etc.), peeled and broken into segments
2 avocados, peeled, pitted, and chopped
½ red onion, minced
¼ cup fresh cilantro leaves
½ cup goat cheese, crumbled (optional)
Lime wedges

1. Set each sweet potato on a plate and sprinkle with a pinch of sea salt and pepper.
2. With a sharp knife, cut a slit down the center. Drizzle in a bit of the vinaigrette. Pile on your preferred toppings and finish with 1-2 tsp. more of the vinaigrette and a squeeze of lime. Serve immediately. *Serves 4*

Marinated Portobello Steaks Stuffed with Spinach
4 large Portobello mushrooms
3 tsp. oregano
2 T. balsamic vinegar
2 T. olive oil
Salt and pepper to taste
2 bags of fresh spinach, chopped
2 T. olive oil
1 cup finely chopped sweet onion (such as Vidalia)
3 garlic cloves, minced
Use mushroom stems from above, chopped
1 x 5 oz. package of goat cheese

1. Cut off stems from mushrooms (and reserve). Brush dirt off mushrooms with a small brush or wipe off with a paper towel. (Never put mushrooms under running water because they will soak it up like a sponge and get soggy.)
2. Blend together next 4 ingredients for marinade.
3. Soak mushrooms in marinade for about an hour (or overnight) in a glass oven proof baking dish. *(cont.)*

4. Add a little water to a skillet and wilt spinach in water until limp. Squeeze out excess water and put spinach in a bowl.
5. Sauté onions in olive oil and when translucent add chopped mushroom stems and garlic. Cook for a few more minutes. Let cool.
6. When ready to cook, preheat oven to 350°F.
7. Drain off marinade.
8. Mix onion mixture into bowl with spinach. Add goat cheese in small chunks.
9. Place a handful of spinach mixture on top of each mushroom.
10. Bake for 20-30 minutes until cheese is somewhat melted.
11. Season with salt and pepper. *Serves 4.*

Asian Tuna Steaks

4 x 6 oz. tuna steaks
1 T. fresh lemon juice
2 T. olive oil
1 cup minced scallion
2 medium cloves garlic, pressed
1 T. minced fresh ginger
2 cups thickly sliced shiitake mushrooms (remove stems)
1 T. chicken broth
1 cup orange juice
2 T. Tamari soy sauce
2 T. cilantro
Salt and pepper to taste

1. Rub tuna with lemon juice and season with a little salt and white pepper.
2. Add olive oil to a really hot frying pan and sear tuna steaks on each side for 2-3 minutes. Set aside (will still be pink in the middle).
3. Heat 1 T. broth in another skillet. Sauté scallion, garlic, ginger and mushrooms in broth for about 2 minutes, stirring constantly over medium heat.
4. Add orange juice and cook for another 2 minutes.
5. Add soy sauce and cilantro.

6. Place tuna on plates and pour mushroom sauce over each piece. Or you can lay a bed of mushroom sauce on each plate and place tuna on top.
7. Serve with Napa Cabbage Salad but omit chicken in recipe. *Serves 4.*

Healthy Cooking Tip:
Because tuna can get dry when cooked it's important to choose very fresh cuts at least 1 inch thick. Tuna is usually best when cooked medium rare. Stick the tip of a sharp knife into it to check for doneness. It should begin to flake on the outside, but still be reddish and firm in the center. Remove it from the heat slightly before it's cooked to your preference, as it continues to cook after it has been removed from the heat.

Garlic Shrimp Salad
4 medium cloves garlic, finely chopped
1 lb. medium-sized cooked shrimp, best bought still frozen
1 bunch asparagus, cut into 1-inch pieces, discarding bottom fourth
3 T. vegetable broth
1 fresh tomato, diced into ½ inch pieces
3 T. chopped fresh parsley (or 3 tsp. dried parsley if fresh not available)
Small head of romaine lettuce, chopped
Salt and fresh cracked black pepper to taste
Optional: 2 oz. crumbled goat cheese

Dressing:
3 T. fresh lemon juice
2 T. extra virgin olive oil
1 T. Dijon mustard
1 tsp. honey
Salt and pepper to taste

1. Finely chop garlic.
2. Make sure shrimp is completely thawed and patted dry with a paper towel, or it will dilute the flavor of the salad.
3. Add broth to medium skillet and after it has heated up, sauté asparagus for 5 minutes. *(cont.)*

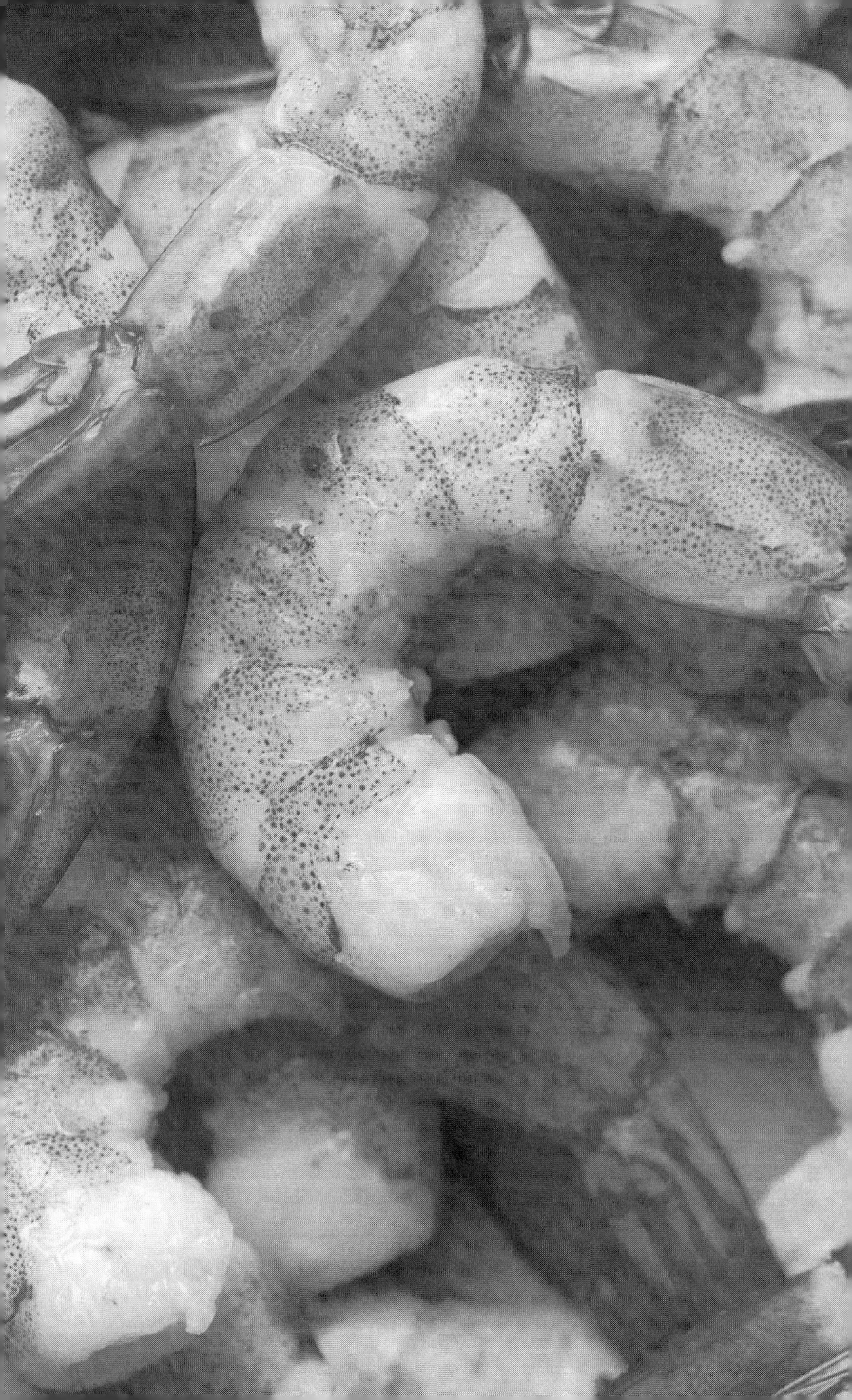

5. Toss shrimp, asparagus, parsley, and tomato with dressing and herbs.
6. Allow shrimp salad to marinate for at least 15 minutes.
7. Discard outer leaves of lettuce head, rinse, dry, and chop.
8. Serve shrimp mixture on a bed of lettuce and top with crumbled goat cheese, if desired. *Serves 4*

Falafel Burgers with Tzatziki

3 cups cooked or canned chickpeas, drained and rinsed
1 small yellow onion, chopped
½ cup flat-leaf parsley
3 T. tahini (sesame paste)
3 T. ground flaxseed
3 garlic cloves, minced, divided
Juice of ½ lemon
¾ tsp. ground cumin
½ tsp. ground coriander
½ tsp. salt
¼ tsp. cayenne, or to taste
Oil, for pan
4 gluten-free buns, optional

<u>Tzatziki</u>
Salt, to sprinkle on cucumbers
½ English cucumber, peeled
¾ cup plain dairy- free yogurt
1 T. chopped mint or dill
2 tsp. olive oil

1. Place chickpeas, onion, parsley, tahini, flaxseed, 2 garlic cloves, lemon juice, cumin, coriander, salt and cayenne in a food processor bowl and blend until slightly grainy. Do not over-blend. (Mixture should not be a smooth paste.) Form into 4 equal-size patties.
2. Lightly coat a skillet with oil and warm over medium heat. Place patties in the pan. Cover and cook 4 minutes per side or until patties are golden brown on top and heated through.
3. Meanwhile, grate the cucumber into a colander. Sprinkle with salt and let stand 5 minutes. Squeeze *(cont.)*

out excess liquid from cucumber. Combine with yogurt, mint, olive oil, remaining garlic and a couple pinches of salt in a small bowl.

4. Serve burgers on buns (if using), topped with tzatziki. *Serves 4*

Vegetable Tofu Stir Fry

1 (14 oz.) package water-packed extra-firm tofu, drained
1 T. organic canola oil, divided
¼ tsp. black pepper
3 ½ tsp. cornstarch, divided
3 large green onions, cut into 1-inch pieces
3 garlic cloves, sliced
1 T. julienne-cut ginger
4 small baby bok choy, quartered lengthwise
2 large carrots, peeled and julienne-cut
1 cup snow peas, trimmed
2 T. rice wine or dry sherry
¼ cup organic vegetable broth
2 T. Tamari soy sauce
1 T. hoisin sauce
1 tsp. dark sesame oil

1. Cut tofu lengthwise into 4 equal pieces; cut each piece crosswise into 1/2-inch squares. Place tofu on several layers of paper towels; cover with additional paper towels. Let stand 30 minutes, pressing down occasionally.
2. Heat a large wok or skillet over high heat. Add 1 ½ teaspoons canola oil to pan; swirl to coat. Combine tofu, pepper, and 2 teaspoons cornstarch in a medium bowl; toss to coat. Add tofu to pan; stir-fry 8 minutes, turning to brown on all sides. Remove tofu from pan with a slotted spoon; place in a medium bowl. Add onions, garlic, and ginger to pan; stir-fry 1 minute. Remove from pan; add to tofu.
3. Add remaining 1 ½ tsp. canola oil to pan; swirl to coat. Add bok choy; stir-fry 3 minutes. Add carrots; stir-fry 2 minutes. Add snow peas; stir-fry 1 minute. Add rice wine, cook 30 seconds, stirring constantly. Stir in tofu mixture.
4. Combine remaining 1 ½ tsp. cornstarch, broth, and remaining ingredients in a small bowl, stirring with a

whisk. Add broth mixture to pan; cook until slightly thickened (about 1 minute).

5. Serve over brown rice. *Serves 4*

Mushroom, Tomato and Basil Frittata

1 T. + 1 T. vegetable broth
½ medium onion, minced
3 medium cloves garlic, finely chopped
1 cup thinly sliced mushrooms
½ medium tomato, seeds removed, diced
3 large eggs
3 T. chopped fresh basil
Salt and black pepper to taste

1. Heat 1 T. broth in a skillet, add onion and sauté over medium low heat for 3 minutes, stirring frequently.
2. Add garlic and mushrooms and continue to sauté for another 2 minutes.
3. Add additional 1 T. broth, tomato, salt and pepper, and cook for another minute.
4. Stir well, and gently scrape pan with a wooden spoon.
5. Beat eggs well, and season with salt and pepper.
6. Mix in chopped basil.
7. Pour eggs over vegetables evenly and turn heat to low. Cover and cook for about 5 minutes, or until firm.
8. Cut into wedges and serve. *Serves 2*

Lemon Ginger Chicken

This moist and flavorful chicken recipe will become a family favorite. Any leftover chicken can be sliced and served cold over lettuce for a quick lunch.

Zest from 1 lemon
1 lemon, juiced (about ¼ cup; use same lemon as above)
2 T. gluten-free soy sauce
½ teaspoon thyme, dried
½ teaspoon oregano, dried
2-4 garlic cloves, sliced
1 tablespoon toasted sesame oil
4-5 fresh ginger slices, rough chopped, approximately 2 tablespoons *(cont.)*

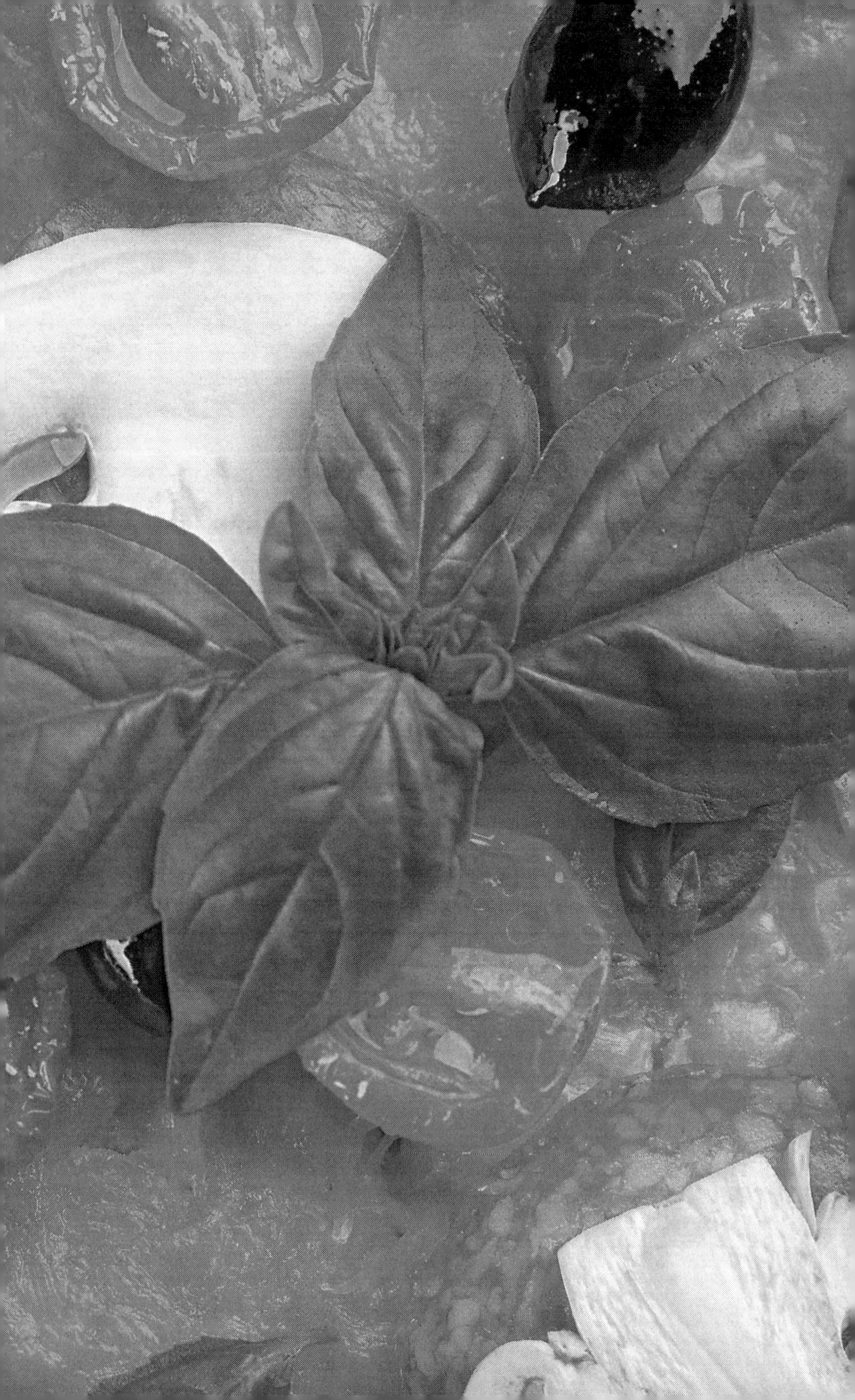

¼ teaspoon fresh ground pepper
4 tablespoons olive oil
8–12 pieces chicken (bone in or boneless)

Additional lemon, sliced thin for serving

1. Remove zest from lemon with a citrus zester, microplane or grater. If you don't have these tools, use a vegetable peeler to carefully remove the zest. Cut the zest into small pieces.
2. Squeeze lemon juice into a bowl with the zest. Add soy sauce, thyme, oregano, garlic, sesame oil, ginger, pepper and olive oil and blend with a whisk.
3. Add chicken pieces, turning them in the marinade several times to coat. Marinate chicken at least 4 hours or overnight in the refrigerator.
4. Preheat grill to medium high. Remove chicken from marinade and discard marinade. Grill chicken until thoroughly cooked.
5. Serve with brown rice and vegetables. *Serves 4-6*

Grilled Halibut with Pomegranate Glaze

2 cups 100% pomegranate juice
1 cup balsamic vinegar
1 tsp. grated orange zest
4 scallions, diced
2 (12 oz.) halibut fillets
1 T. olive oil
¼ tsp. sea salt to taste
½ tsp. black pepper

1. Bring juice and vinegar to a boil in a small saucepan over high heat.
2. Reduce heat to medium and let simmer, uncovered until reduced by half (about 15 min).
3. Mix in orange zest and scallions.
4. Pour ¾ of glaze into separate bowl and set aside. Keep remaining ¼ of glaze in a small pitcher.
5. Preheat grill.
6. Rinse halibut with cold water and pat dry with paper towel. *(cont.)*

7. Rub oil on both sides and season with salt and pepper.
8. Grill on one side for 4-5 minutes.
9. Flip fish and brush on half of glaze from bowl. Continue to cook for another 4-5 minutes until opaque in center.
10. Transfer to a serving plate and brush with other half of glaze.
11. Serve immediately with remaining glaze in the small pitcher on the side. *Serves 2*

Note: You can serve with Millet Pilaf recipe or brown rice and grilled zucchini.

Lentil Shephard's Pie

1 onion, finely diced
2 carrots, finely diced
½ cup sweet peas (frozen are fine)
1 stalk of celery, finely diced
1 can of organic corn
1 large can of lentils (or 1 cup dried lentils, cooked)
5–7 large Yukon gold potatoes
¼ cup rice milk
Sea salt and pepper to taste
Pinch of cumin
½ tsp. thyme
2 T. Tamari soy sauce
1 tsp. dried paprika
Oil for cooking

1. In a large pot, cook the peeled potatoes in salted water.
2. In a large pan, saute the chopped onions, carrots, celery – cook until golden, add the frozen peas and lentils and cover to cook for a few minutes. Add a bit of water if these veggies start to stick to the bottom of the pan.
3. Add in the corn and Tamari, and season with cumin and thyme, salt and pepper. Keep covered, turn down the heat to low.
4. The potatoes should be boiled by now. Drain them, leaving some of the water near the bottom. Mash the potatoes with the rice milk until a puree forms. Taste and season with salt and pepper.

5. In an oven-safe dish, place in the whole mix of vegetables with lentils into the bottom of the pan and spread out evenly. Add the mashed potatoes on top and smooth out over top with the back of the spoon. Sprinkle the top with dried paprika, and poke through with a fork to make vents in the mashed potatoes. Bake at 350°F for 20-30 minutes. Let it set for 10 minutes before serving, but serve while still hot. *Serves 6-8*

SIDE DISHES

Sautéed Escarole with Sundried Tomatoes

Note: Escarole is also known as broad-leaved endive. Look for broad heads with dark green leaves, available year-round.

1/3 cup sundried tomatoes (not packed in oil), thinly sliced
¼ cup boiling water
1 T. olive oil
3 cloves garlic, smashed with side of chef's knife
1 large head escarole (1¾ lbs.), coarsely chopped
Salt and pepper

1. Place tomatoes in small bowl.
2. Cover with boiling water and let stand 5 minutes to rehydrate.
3. Pour off any remaining water if necessary.
4. Meanwhile, in deep 12-inch skillet, heat olive oil on medium until hot.
5. Add garlic and cook 1 minute, stirring.
6. Increase heat to high; gradually add escarole, tomatoes, ½ tsp. salt, and ¼ tsp. coarsely ground black pepper, and cook about 8 minutes or until escarole wilts, stirring constantly. *Serves 6*

Creamy Sesame Greens

This simple side dish pairs your favorite greens with tahini, lemon juice and garlic.

4 T. water
6 cups chopped kale, Swiss chard or collard greens, tough stems removed
2 T. tahini
2 T. orange or lemon juice
1 clove garlic, finely chopped

1. Heat 2 T. water in a large skillet over medium heat.
2. Add greens and cook, tossing occasionally, until wilted, about 5 minutes.

3. Drain well.
4. In a large bowl, whisk together tahini, orange juice, remaining 2 T. water and garlic.
5. Add hot greens, toss to combine and serve immediately. *Serves 2*

Creamed Kale

½ cup vegetable broth
1 onion, finely chopped
1 cup unsweetened soy milk or other nondairy milk
¼ cup raw cashews
1 tsp. onion powder
1 tsp. mellow white miso
Pinch of freshly grated nutmeg
Pinch of red pepper flakes
4 cups chopped kale or other dark, leafy green

1. Heat broth in a large skillet over medium heat.
2. Add onion and cook until softened, 5 to 7 minutes.
3. Transfer to a blender or food processor.
4. Add soy milk, cashews, onion powder, miso, nutmeg and pepper flakes and purée until smooth.
5. Transfer blended mixture back to skillet and bring to simmer over medium heat.
6. Stir in kale and continue simmering, tossing often until kale is just tender, about 5 minutes.

Baked Parmesan Tomatoes

4 medium tomatoes, halved horizontally
¼ cup grated Vegan parmesan cheese
1 tsp. oregano, fresh, chopped
¼ tsp. salt
Black pepper, ground to taste
4 tsp. olive oil

1. Preheat oven to 450°F.
2. Spray cookie sheet and place tomatoes cut-side up on the sheet.
3. Top with parmesan cheese, oregano, salt and pepper.
4. Bake until the tomatoes are tender, about 15-20 minutes. *Serves 4*

Fennel with Raisins and Pine Nuts

Note: Be sure to remove the fennel's core entirely, so the slices will separate easily.

3 T. pine nuts
½ cup golden raisins
¾ cup water, divided
2 fennel bulbs (about 2 lbs.)
2 T. extra-virgin olive oil
1 small onion, finely chopped
1 tsp. balsamic vinegar
¼ tsp. salt, or to taste
½ tsp. freshly ground pepper

1. In a large nonstick skillet, heat the pine nuts over medium heat until toasted, about 4 minutes. Transfer to a bowl and set aside.
2. Place raisins in a small bowl. Bring ½ cup of the water to a boil and pour over the raisins. Set aside.
3. Trim stems from fennel bulb. Remove the fronds from the stems and chop 2 T. of fronds for garnish. Discard stems and any remaining fronds.
4. Cut bulbs in half. Cut out the cores, then slice fennel into ¼ inch thick slices.
5. Add to a large nonstick skillet or saucepan with remaining ¼ cup water and oil. Bring to a boil over medium-high heat. Cover pan and cook, shaking the pan occasionally, until fennel is just barely tender, about 3 to 4 minutes.
6. Uncover, add onion, and continue to cook, stirring occasionally, until the liquid evaporates and the fennel begins to sizzle in the oil, about 2 minutes.
7. Drain the raisins, discard the soaking liquid, and add to fennel. Continue to cook, stirring constantly, until fennel is tender, about 2 to 4 minutes longer.
8. Add vinegar, salt, pepper, toasted pine nuts, and reserved fennel fronds, and toss to distribute.
9. Transfer to a platter and serve immediately. *Serves 6*

Millet Pilaf with Almonds and Feta
2 T. extra-virgin olive oil
4 scallions, thinly sliced, white and green portions separated
2 cups cooked and cooled millet
1/3 cup toasted slivered almonds
4 oz. feta crumbles
¼ cup finely chopped parsley
¼ tsp. each salt and pepper
Lemon wedges, for serving

1. In a medium skillet, add 2 T. extra-virgin olive oil and the thinly sliced white portions of the scallions and cook, stirring, for 2 minutes.
2. Stir in the thinly sliced green portions of the scallions, then transfer to a large bowl with cooled millet, feta crumbles, almonds, parsley and ¼ tsp. each salt and pepper.
3. Serve with lemon wedges. *Serves 4*

7-Minute Butternut Squash
2 cups butternut squash, or any variety of winter squash, cut into 1-inch cubes
3 T. extra virgin olive oil
1 tsp. orange juice
Sea salt and pepper to taste
Optional: feta cheese, chopped fresh rosemary, ½ small onion sliced thin, cooked with the squash

1. Fill the bottom of a steamer with 2 inches of water.
2. While steam is building up in steamer, peel and cut squash into 1-inch cubes. Steam, covered for 7 minutes. Squash is done when it is tender, yet still firm enough to hold its shape. Transfer to a bowl.
3. Toss squash with the oil, orange juice, salt, and pepper while it is still hot. Research shows that carotenoids in foods are best absorbed when consumed with oils.
Serves 2

Note: Also try combining 4 tsp. finely minced fresh ginger, ½ tsp. cinnamon and 2 tsp. honey with the olive oil.

Bok Choy with Sesame Orange Dressing

1 lb. baby Bok Choy, separate white parts from green parts and diced
2 T. oil
8 ounces shiitake mushrooms, stemmed and sliced
4 medium carrots, shredded
2 T. orange juice
1 T. tahini
1 ½ tsp. gluten free soy sauce
½ tsp. grated fresh ginger
1 T. toasted sesame seeds

1. Sauté white parts of Bok Choy in oil for 3 minutes.
2. Add carrots and mushrooms and continue sautéing for another 3-4 minutes.
3. Add in green parts of Bok Choy and sauté until wilted.
4. In a large bowl, whisk together orange juice, tahini, Tamari and ginger.
5. Add Bok Choy, mushrooms, and carrots and toss to coat. Garnish with sesame seeds. *Serves 4*

Root Fries with Gremolata

2 lbs. of root vegetables in whatever combination you like: potatoes, sweet potatoes, carrots, yams, rutabagas, and parsnips
4 T. olive oil
2 T. chopped fresh sage leaves (or 2 tsp. dried sage)
Sea salt
2 T. finely chopped parsley
2 garlic cloves, minced
1 tsp. finely grated lemon zest

1. Preheat oven to 400°F.
2. Peel the vegetables and cut into 3-inch batons that are between ½ and ¾ inch thick. Place in a bowl and add olive oil; toss until evenly coated. Season with sage and salt.
3. Transfer to a large roasting pan. Roast for 20 minutes, stir well, and then continue roasting until crispy on the outside and tender inside, about 40 minutes total.
4. Toss with parsley, garlic, and lemon zest. *Serves 4-6*

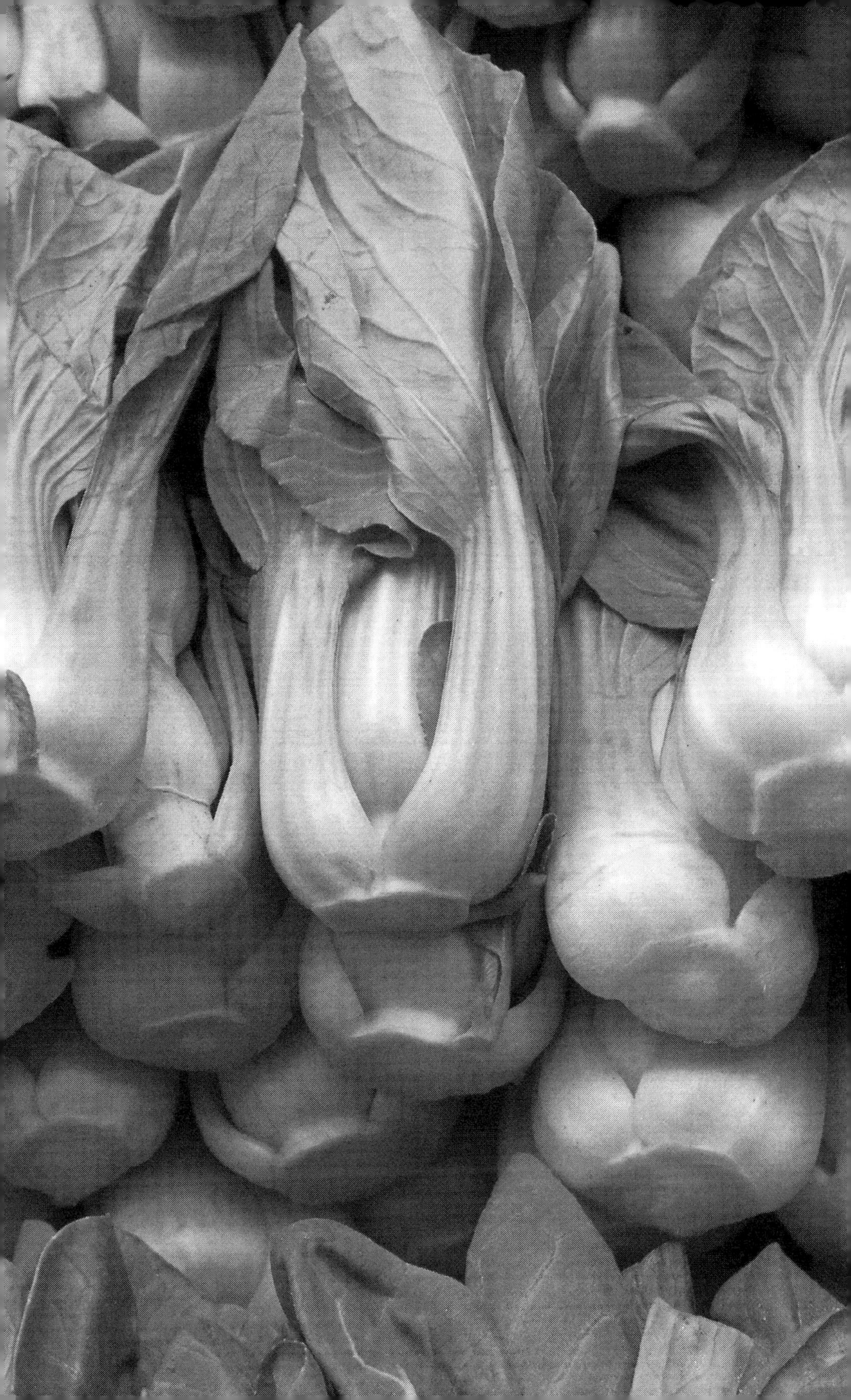

Calabacitas (Mexican-flavored vegetable side dish)
This recipe is an excellent source of health-promoting vitamin C, a powerful antioxidant that helps prevent damage to DNA and cellular structures caused by free radicals.

1 medium onion, cut in half and sliced thin
4 medium cloves garlic, chopped
2 cups zucchini, diced into ½ inch cubes
2 cups yellow squash, diced in ½ inch cubes
15 oz. can diced tomatoes, drained
4 oz. can of diced green chili
1 T. + 3 T. chicken or vegetable broth
¼ cup chopped cilantro
3 T. fresh chopped fresh oregano (or 1 T. dried oregano)
Salt and black pepper to taste

1. Slice onion and chop garlic and let sit for at least 5 minutes to bring out their health-promoting benefits.
2. Prepare all the vegetables.
3. Heat 1 T. broth in a 12 inch stainless steel skillet. Sauté onions in broth over medium heat for about 5 minutes stirring frequently, until translucent.
4. Add garlic and sauté for another minute.
5. Add zucchini, yellow squash, remaining broth, green chili, and cook for another 3 minutes or so until vegetables are tender, stirring often.
6. Add tomatoes and continue to cook for another couple of minutes.
7. Stir in herbs, salt, and pepper. Optional: drizzle with olive oil before serving. *Serves 4*

Healthy Cooking Tip:
Have all your vegetables cut before you start cooking to avoid overcooking. The zucchini will start to look translucent and will release a lot of water, diluting the flavor of your dish if it is overcooked.

Roasted Radishes and Leeks

2 bunches radishes (about 1 pound), halved if small, quartered if large
1 T. extra-virgin olive oil
½ tsp. salt
¼ tsp. freshly ground pepper
1 large leek, white and light green part only, halved and thinly sliced
1 T. coconut oil
1 tsp. finely chopped fresh thyme or ¼ tsp. dried

1. Preheat oven to 450°F.
2. Combine radishes, oil, salt and pepper in a large roasting pan and roast for 10 minutes.
3. Stir in leek. Continue roasting until the radishes are lightly browned and tender, 10 to 15 minutes more. Stir in butter and thyme; serve warm. *Serves 4*

Garlic Gingered Broccoli

1 bunch broccoli
3 cloves garlic, minced
6 cups water
1 T. olive oil
2 T. Tamari soy sauce
4 inch piece fresh ginger, finely grated
Tarragon or basil for garnish (optional)

1. Wash and cut broccoli into florets. Peel stems and cut into ½ inch pieces.
2. Add water to large pot and boil.
3. Add broccoli and quick boil for 3 minutes.
4. Drain and rinse quickly in cold water.
5. Heat skillet with oil, add garlic and sauté for a few seconds before adding broccoli. Sauté broccoli and garlic for a few more minutes then add soy sauce and ginger.
6. Sauté a few more minutes until tender. *Serves 4*

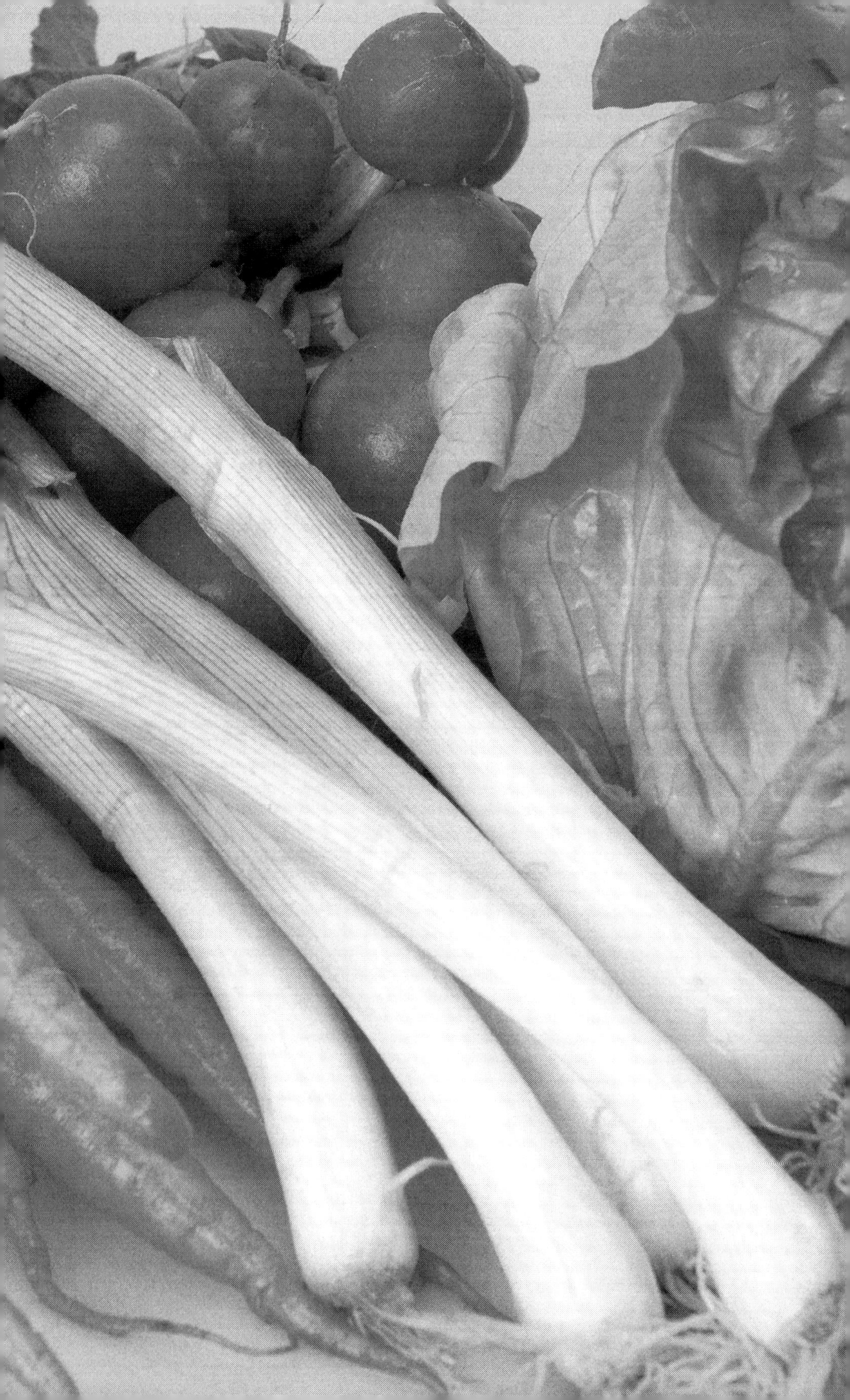

Apple Beet Relish
3 large apples, cored but not peeled
3 large beets, peeled
2 star anise pods
1 T. whole cloves
1 T. sea salt
Fermented vegetable starter culture (or substitute another T. of sea salt)

1. Shred apples and beets by hand, or in a food processor. Mix the shredded apples and beets together until well combined.
2. Add the star anise and whole cloves to the apples and beetroot, and continue to toss until the spices are evenly distributed among the shredded fruit and vegetables.
3. In a mason jar, layer the apple and beetroot.
4. Periodically sprinkle the sea salt or vegetable starter culture over the layers of apple and beetroot and mash with a wooden spoon or mallet to encourage the fruit and vegetables to release their juices, creating a luscious brine to encourage the proliferation of beneficial bacteria.
5. Put on the lid and ferment for a minimum of three to four days, or longer, depending on the level of warmth in your kitchen.
6. After your apple and beetroot relish has sufficiently cultured, gently pick out the star anise pods and whole cloves.
7. Place the apple and beetroot relish into a blender or food processor and process until smooth.
   Yields approximately 48 oz.

SOUPS

Easy Broccoli Soup
2 broccoli heads and most of the stem
(washed and roughly chopped)
4-6 cloves of garlic – whole
3 T. olive oil
1 cup of vegetable stock (or water)
Salt to taste
½ tsp. onion powder

1. Wash and roughly chop broccoli
(trim the woody part of the stem; use the rest).
2. Add broccoli florets, stems, and peeled garlic to a baking dish.
3. Coat with olive oil and add some salt.
4. Roast in oven for about 15 minutes.
5. Remove from oven and transfer to a blender or food processor.
6. Add in vegetable stock or water, salt to taste, and onion powder.
7. Blend until smooth.
8. Garnish with parsley or eat just as it is. *Serves 4*

Hearty Greens Soup
Use any manner of hearty greens in this filling soup.

6. 4 T. olive oil
3 cloves garlic, chopped
1 medium yellow onion, chopped
1 bay leaf
Salt and pepper to taste
4 plum tomatoes, cored and chopped
2 carrots, chopped
8 cups water
1 bunch Swiss chard (about ¾ lb.), roughly chopped
½ bunch escarole (about ½ lb.), stemmed and roughly chopped

(cont.)

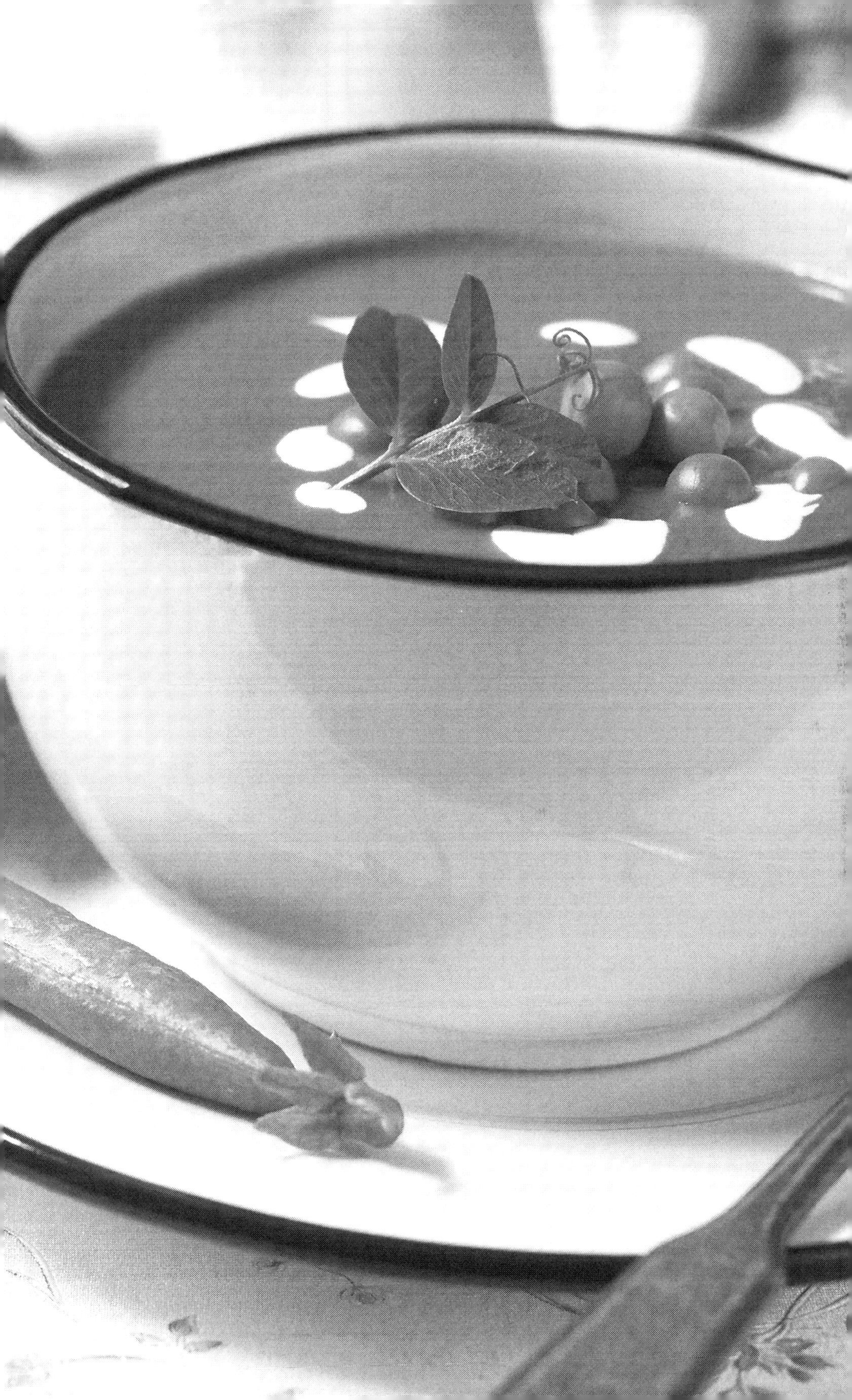

½ lb. gluten free bowtie (farfalle) pasta
¼ lb. baby spinach

1. Heat oil in a large pot over medium heat.
2. Add garlic, onions, bay leaf, salt and pepper and cook, stirring often, until caramelized, about 15 minutes.
3. Add tomatoes and cook until most of the liquid is released and absorbed, about 5 minutes more.
4. Add carrots and water and bring to a boil, scraping up any browned bits from the bottom of the pot.
5. Stir in Swiss chard, escarole and pasta.
6. Reduce heat, cover and simmer until broth is flavorful and greens and pasta are tender, about 15 minutes.
7. Stir in spinach and season with salt and pepper.
8. Remove and discard bay leaf from soup, ladle into bowls and serve. *Serves 6-8*

Fresh Pea Soup

I use organic frozen peas to make this beautiful bright-green soup. Adding them to the pot at the tail end of the cooking time preserves their sweet flavor and vivid green color.

2 T. butter
1 leek, trimmed, washed and sliced
1 russet potato, peeled and cut into small pieces
4 cups chicken broth
2 lb. (6 cups) frozen peas
Salt and pepper

1. Melt the butter in a medium pot over medium heat.
2. Add the leeks and cook, stirring often, until soft but not colored, about 10 minutes.
3. Add the potatoes and chicken broth to the pot and cook until the potatoes are tender, about 20 minutes.
4. Add the peas and season with some salt and pepper. When the peas are heated through, about 3 minutes, remove the pot from the heat.
5. Working in batches, puree the soup in a blender. For a smoother texture, pass it through a strainer into a bowl, discarding the solids.

6. Taste the soup and season it with more salt, if you like, as it will probably need it.
7. Return the soup to the pot and warm it over low heat. Or, cover and refrigerate it until cold. *Makes 6 cups*

Golden Squash Soup

1 medium-sized butternut squash, peeled and cut into ½ inch pieces (about 3 cups)
1 large onion, chopped
3 medium cloves garlic, chopped
1 T. chopped fresh ginger
1 tsp. turmeric
1 tsp. curry powder
1T. + 2¾ cups chicken or vegetable broth
6 oz. canned coconut milk
2 T. chopped fresh cilantro
Salt and white pepper to taste

1. Chop onion and garlic. Peel and cut squash.
2. Heat 1 T. broth in medium soup pot. Sauté onion in broth over medium heat for about 5 minutes, stirring frequently, until translucent.
3. Add garlic and ginger, and continue to sauté for another minute.
4. Add turmeric and curry powder, and mix well. Add squash and broth, and mix. Bring to a boil on high heat.
5. Once it comes to a boil, reduce heat to medium-low and simmer uncovered until squash is tender, about 10 minutes.
6. Place in blender and blend with coconut milk. Make sure you blend in batches, filling blender only half full. Start on low speed, so hot soup does not erupt and burn you. Blend until smooth, about 1 minute.
7. Thin with a little broth if needed.
8. Season to taste with salt and white pepper.
9. Reheat and add cilantro. *Serves 4*

Tomato Basil Soup

4 large ripe tomatoes
1 tsp. garlic powder
7. ¾ cup extra virgin olive oil *(cont.)*

2 tsp. sea salt
Fresh basil, sliced fine for garnish

1. Blend everything together in a blender or food processor except the basil.
2. Sprinkle sliced basil on top and enjoy cold. *Serves 2*

Creamy Radish Soup

2 T. extra-virgin olive oil
2 cups sliced radishes (from 2 bunches), divided
½ cup chopped onion
1 medium Yukon Gold potato (about 8 ounces), peeled and cut into 1-inch cubes
2 cups coconut milk
½ tsp. salt
¼ tsp. white or black pepper
Garnish with chives

1. Heat oil in a large saucepan over medium-high heat. Add 1 ¾ cups radishes and onion and cook, stirring frequently, until the onions are beginning to brown and the radishes are translucent, about 5 minutes.
2. Add potato, milk, salt and pepper to taste. Bring to a boil, stirring occasionally.
3. Reduce heat to a simmer, cover and cook, stirring occasionally, until the potato is tender, about 5 minutes more.
4. Working in batches, puree the mixture in a blender (or in the pan with an immersion blender) until smooth. (Use caution when pureeing hot liquids.)
5. Slice the remaining ¼ cup radishes into matchsticks. Serve each portion of soup topped with some radish matchsticks and a sprinkling of chives. *Serves 4*

Artichoke Leek Soup

2 T. olive oil
2 medium leeks, white part only, chopped (2 cups)
9 cloves garlic, peeled
2 cups vegetable broth
1 9.9 oz. jar water-packed artichoke hearts, rinsed and

drained or 1 10 oz. bag frozen artichoke hearts, thawed
2 medium boiling potatoes, peeled and cut into 1 inch pieces
6 fresh thyme sprigs or 1 ½ tsp. dried thyme
2 tsp. fresh lemon juice
6 T. prepared basil pesto

1. Heat oil in large skillet over medium heat.
2. Add leeks and garlic and sauté for 5 minutes or until leeks are softened and translucent.
3. Add broth, artichokes, potatoes, thyme and 2 cups of water. Cover and bring to a boil.
4. Reduce heat to medium low, season with salt and pepper, if desired, and simmer, partially covered for 20-25 minutes.
5. Remove thyme sprigs (if using) and strip remaining thyme leaves into the soup pot.
6. Transfer the soup to a blender or food processor and blend until smooth.
7. Return to pot and stir in lemon juice.
8. Season again with salt and pepper, if desired.
9. Garnish each serving with 1 T. prepared pesto. *Serves 6*

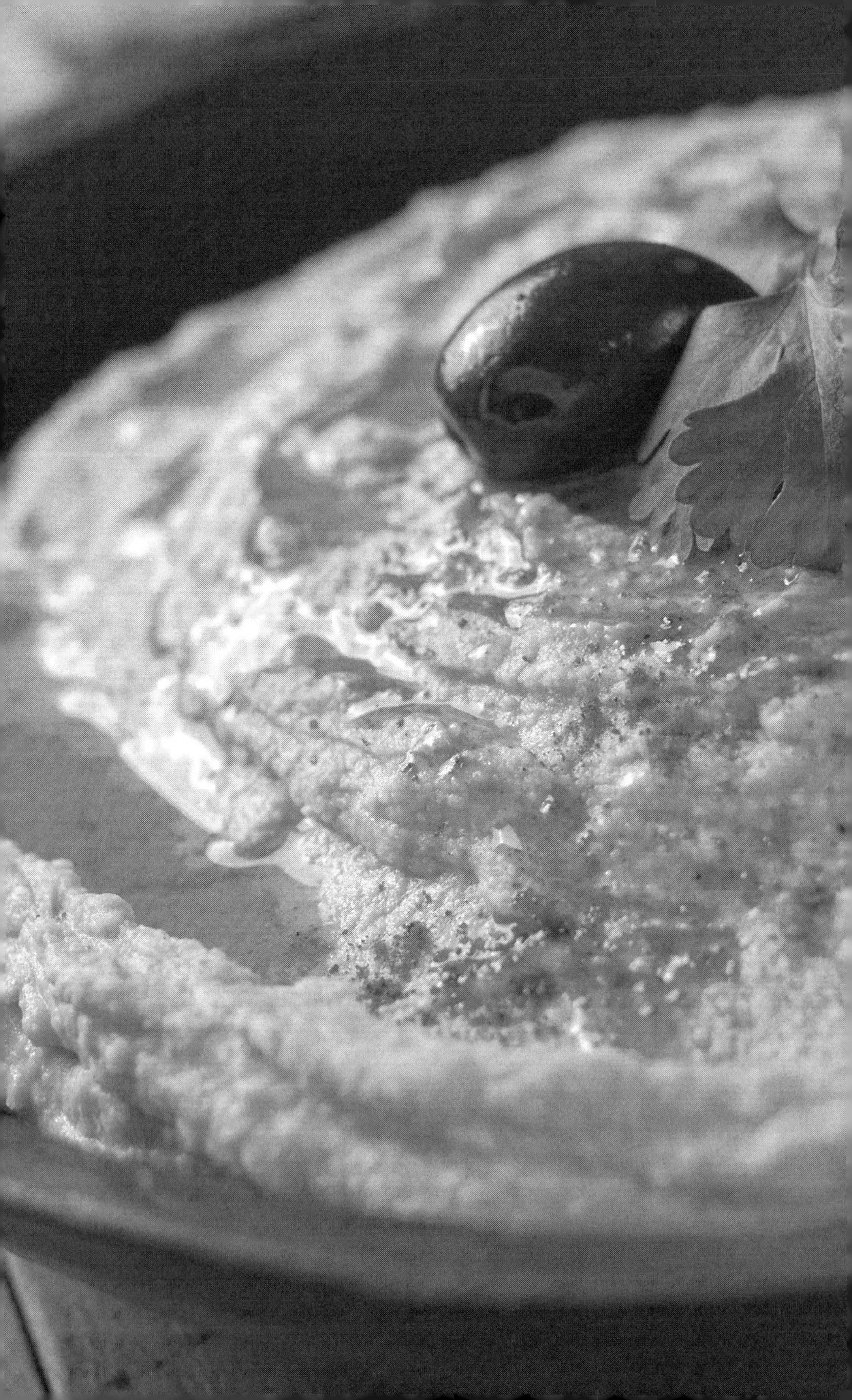

SNACKS

Hummus
2 cups cooked dried chickpeas (or canned)
½ cup tahini
¼ cup extra virgin olive oil
2 cloves garlic, peeled
Juice of 1 big or 2 small lemons, plus zest
Salt and pepper to taste

1. In a blender or food processor, add all ingredients and blend until smooth.
2. Taste and adjust seasonings.
3. Add water as needed to create smooth consistency.
4. Serve with cucumber slices, celery sticks and carrots.

Raw Granola Bars
½ cup honey
¼ cup coconut oil
¼ cup organic peanut butter
1 tsp. vanilla extract
1 cup rolled gluten free oats
½ cup raw almonds, coarsely chopped
¼ cup raw sunflower seeds
¼ cup raw pumpkin seeds
¼ cup raw pistachios
¼ cup raw macadamia nuts
¼ cup cashews, coarsely chopped

1. Place first four wet ingredients together in a small pan and heat on low until melted together. Mix the remaining dry ingredients in a large bowl.
2. Add the wet ingredients to the dry ingredients, blend well.
3. Press mixture into a 9 x 9 inch pan and refrigerate.
4. Cut into bars and enjoy!

You can freeze these for later use.
Makes about 6-8 depending on how big you cut them.

(cont.)

You can replace ¼ cup of any of the nuts with unsweetened coconut flakes or raw cacao nibs for a chocolaty taste!

Spiced Popcorn
½ tsp. ground cumin
½ tsp. chili powder
¼ tsp. salt
Dash cayenne pepper
Dash cinnamon
12 cups air-popped popcorn
Cooking spray

1. In a small bowl, stir together cumin, chili powder, salt, cayenne pepper, and cinnamon. Spread popped popcorn in an even layer in a large shallow baking pan.
2. Lightly coat popcorn with nonstick cooking spray.
3. Sprinkle the cumin mixture evenly over popcorn; toss to coat.

Tip: Indian Spiced Popcorn: Prepare Spiced Popcorn as directed, except substitute ½ tsp. curry powder, ½ tsp. garam masala, ¼ tsp. ground turmeric, and ¼ tsp. ground black pepper for the cumin, chili powder, cayenne pepper, and cinnamon.

Sesame Kale Chips
1 head of kale
2 T. toasted sesame oil
1 T. umeboshi plum vinegar
2 T. sesame seeds

1. Rinse kale leaves and shake dry.
2. Tear leaves into bite-size pieces.
3. In a large bowl, combine kale with oil, vinegar and sesame seeds. Mix with your hands – it's easier.
4. Preheat oven to 350°F.
5. Spread kale out on two large baking sheets covered with foil so they are not overlapping. Grind fresh black pepper over them.
6. Bake for about 7 minutes.

7. Flip and move chips around to cook evenly.
8. Bake another 7 minutes or so until crispy. Careful not to overcook or burn; it happens fast! Serve immediately.

If you prefer simpler ingredients, olive oil with salt and pepper also does the trick!

Tuscan White Bean Dip

1½ cups cooked dried great northern beans or one 15 oz. can, drained
¼ cup pine nuts
2 cloves garlic, minced
½ tsp. salt or to taste
1 T. balsamic vinegar
1 T. fresh, minced rosemary
¼ cup sundried tomatoes, soaked in lukewarm water until soft (about 1 hour), then minced (or sundried tomatoes in oil – drained and no need for soaking)

1. Place all ingredients, except the sundried tomatoes, in a high-powered blender or a food processor. Process until smooth and creamy.
2. Adjust seasonings to taste. Stir in the sundried tomatoes.
3. Chill for one hour before serving.
4. Serve topped with an extra drizzle of balsamic vinegar and a sprinkle of pine nuts.
5. Enjoy with raw vegetables. *Serves 5*

Homemade Ginger Tea

If you are feeling tired, weepy or just want to cry, this tea is an amazing way to comfort yourself. It helps calm you down during stressful situations and just generally mellows your mood!

1 T. freshly grated ginger
4 cups water
1 T. raw agave nectar

1. Take a whole ginger root and peel about an inch.
2. Holding the unpeeled portion, run the peeled part through a cheese grater or a micro-plane. *(cont.)*

3. Place ginger in a teapot. Bring water to a boil and pour over ginger.
4. Let steep for several minutes and then stir in agave nectar or stevia.
5. Strain into teacups.

Serves 4; if you want just one cup for yourself, cut everything to ¼

Guacamole (RAW)
2 ripe avocados
1 ripe medium tomato
2 T. fresh cilantro, minced
1 T. onion, minced
Juice of 1 lime
Sprinkle of cumin (optional)

1. Peel and pit the avocados and place in a big bowl. Mash with a fork.
2. Dice the tomato and onion and add to the bowl.
3. Add the cilantro, lime juice and cumin and continue to mash or use your hands to work it. You can keep it in the refrigerator for several hours to allow the flavors to combine or serve immediately with romaine lettuce leaves and sprouts or on celery sticks.
   Yields approx. 1½ cups

Cucumber Pizzas (RAW)
This is a simple appetizer. The saltiness of the olives makes the cucumber stand out.
3 seedless English cucumbers, sliced in to rounds
2 cups chopped green and black olives

1. Arrange the cucumber slices on an attractive platter.
2. Top with chopped olives and serve.
3. You can add a drizzle of extra virgin olive oil if you like.
   Serves 12 for a party

Parmesan Pita Crisps
2 T. grated non-dairy parmesan cheese (or raw cashew 'uncheese')
4-inch gluten free pita

¼ tsp. dried oregano

1. Sprinkle grated parmesan evenly over pita.
2. Dust pita with oregano and broil until the cheese browns. Cut into quarters. *Serves 1*

Roasted Red Pepper Almond Dip
1 cup roasted red peppers
1 small plum tomato, seeded
¼ cup almonds
1 garlic clove
2 T. extra virgin olive oil
1 tsp. paprika

1. In a food processor, combine roasted red peppers, tomato, almonds, garlic, oil, and paprika and puree until smooth.
2. Season with salt.

Healthy Ants on a Log
2 celery sticks
3 T. cashew butter
Handful of golden raisins

1. Spread cashew butter on celery stick and dot with raisins.

Elegant Endive
4 endive lettuce spears
1 bosc pear
Balsamic vinegar

1. Break off 4 spears of endive lettuce from main head.
2. Peel and slice the ripe pear.
3. Place a few slices in each spear.
4. Drizzle with the vinegar.

Instant California Roll
1 ripe avocado
Small can of tuna fish or lump crab meat
A dash of wasabi *(cont.)*

1 T. soy sauce

1. Quarter a ripe avocado and remove the pit.
2. Mix the wasabi paste and soy sauce in a small bowl.
3. Stuff the avocado holes with the tuna or crab and drizzle with soy sauce mix.

Five-Spice Pumpkin Seeds
1 cup pumpkin seeds
1 T. sesame oil
¼ tsp. Chinese five spice powder

1. Toss salted pumpkin seeds (also known as pepitas) with sesame oil and chinese five-spice powder.
2. Bake at 350°F on a foil lined cookie sheet until crisp.

DESSERTS

Apple Pumpkin Spice Cake
5 medjool dates, pitted
¼ cup warm water
¾ cup pumpkin puree
1 ¼ cups diced unpeeled apples, divided
¼ cup coconut oil
3 eggs
2 cups almond flour
¼ cup coconut flour
1 tsp. cinnamon
1 tsp. nutmeg
½ tsp. cloves
½ tsp. allspice
1 ½ tsp. vanilla extract
1 tsp. baking soda
½ tsp. salt

1. Preheat oven to 350°F.
2. In a food processor, combine dates with water.
3. Let them sit for a few minutes to soften.
4. Then add pumpkin, ¾ cup diced apples, coconut oil and eggs.
5. Blend very well.
6. Transfer to a large mixing bowl.
7. Add flours, spices, vanilla, baking soda and salt.
8. Mix well to combine.
9. Pour batter into a greased loaf pan.
10. Top with remaining ½ cup diced apples.
11. Bake for 45-50 minutes.
12. Cool before slicing. *Serves 6*

Chia Cream
4 T. chia seeds
¾ cup coconut milk
Generous amount of: dried fruits, nuts, shredded coconut, cocoa, cinnamon, etc.

1. In a bowl, combine seeds with coconut milk.

2. Stir well.
3. Let mixture sit for 30 minutes.
4. Stir every 5–10 minutes. The consistency will become thick like tapioca pudding. You may want to refrigerate at this point for a cool treat.
5. Add toppings and enjoy. *Serves 2*

Apple Bread Pudding

4 cups of ½ inch gluten free bread cubes
1 cup finely chopped apple pieces
¼ cup chopped walnuts
¾ tsp. cinnamon
¼ tsp. nutmeg
¼ tsp. salt
2 cups plain almond milk
1/3 cup and 1 T. agave nectar or maple syrup, plus more for drizzling

1. Preheat the oven to 350°F.
2. Lightly oil two 2-cup heatproof dishes or, alternately, six 6-ounce ramekins.
3. Set aside.
4. In a medium-sized bowl, combine the bread cubes, apple pieces, walnuts, cinnamon, nutmeg and salt until well mixed
5. Using a wooden spoon, stir in the almond milk and agave nectar and allow the mixture to stand for 10 minutes.
6. Portion the mixture into the prepared dishes and bake until golden brown, about 30-35 minutes. (If baking ramekin-sized puddings, bake for 15-20 minutes.)
7. Drizzle with syrup and serve warm.

Makes two 2-cup puddings or six 6-oz ramekin puddings

Chocolate Cherry Cookies

2 ½ cups blanched almond flour
½ tsp. salt
½ tsp. baking soda
¼ cup. raw cacao powder
½ cup coconut oil (coconut butter is even better!)
¾ cup raw agave nectar

1 T. vanilla extract
1 cup coarsely chopped dark chocolate (as high a % of cacao as you can stand)
1 cup fruit-juice-sweetened dried cherries

1. Preheat oven to 350°F.
2. Line 2 large baking sheets with parchment paper.
3. In a large mixing bowl, combine almond flour, salt, baking soda and raw cacao powder.
4. In a medium bowl, whisk together the oil, agave, and vanilla.
5. Fold the wet ingredients into the almond flour mixture until thoroughly combined.
6. Stir in chocolate and cherries.
7. Spoon the dough (1 heaping T. at a time) onto the prepared baking sheet, leaving 2 inches between each cookie.
8. Bake for 10-15 minutes, until the tops of the cookies look dry and start to crack—be careful not to overcook.
9. Let the cookies cool on the baking sheet for 20 minutes, then serve warm. *Makes 2 dozen*

Fried Peanut Butter Bananas
1 T. butter
1 banana, sliced thick
1½ T. natural peanut butter (only ingredients are peanuts and salt)
⅛ tsp. unsweetened baking cocoa (raw cacao)

1. In a small pan, heat butter over medium-high heat.
2. Add banana slices and cook for a minute or two on each side. Transfer bananas to plate.
3. In the same pan, reduce heat to low and combine peanut butter and cocoa powder. Stir until melted and pour over bananas. *Serves 1*

Cranberry and Fresh Pear Cobbler
1 medium orange
½ cup dried cranberries
2 tsp. honey *(cont.)*

½ ripe pear (Bosc or other firm variety)
¼ cup + 2 T. walnuts

1. Grate enough orange rind to make 1 tsp. zest and place in a mixing bowl.
2. Cut the orange in half and juice both halves into the same bowl as the rind.
3. Add the cranberries and honey. Mix until the honey is dissolved. Let sit for ½ hour to allow cranberries to soften.
4. After the cranberries have softened, cut the pear into ¼ inch cubes and add to the bowl.
5. Add ¼ cup walnuts.
6. Divide the mixture into 2 dessert dishes and sprinkle each with 1 T. of the chopped walnuts. *Serves 2*

Chocolate Chia Pudding

1 can full fat coconut milk
4 T. chia seeds
4 T. raw cacao
¼ tsp. Stevia Powder or 2 T. honey or maple syrup
½ tsp. gluten free vanilla extract

1. Mix the coconut milk and the cacao powder until dissolved.
2. Add the chia, vanilla, sweetener, and mix well.
3. Put it in the freezer for 10 minutes.
4. Eat and Enjoy. *Serves 3*

Cantaloupe Mint Paletas (Ice Pops)

Equipment: Popsicle molds or can use Dixie cups with foil over them and a popsicle stick inserted in center.

2 cups cantaloupe, peeled, seeded and cut into chunks
¼ cup freshly squeezed lime juice
2 tsp. honey (optional)
Pinch of sea salt
1 T. fresh mint leaves, chopped

1. Place the cantaloupe, lime juice, honey and sea salt in a blender or food processor. Blend until smooth.

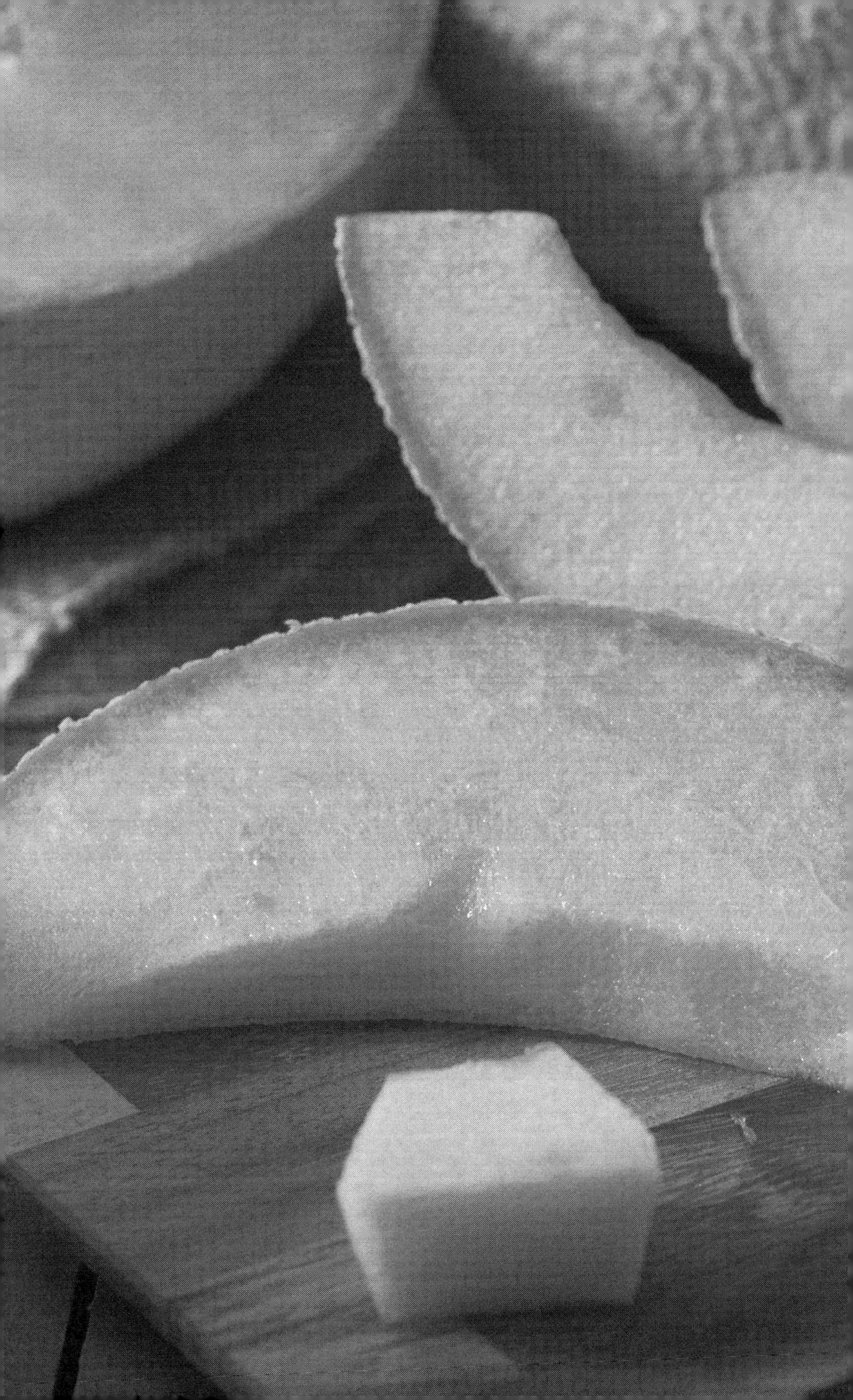

2. Add mint and pulse for a few more seconds, until it is combined into the cantaloupe mixture.
3. Pour cantaloupe mixture into popsicle molds or Dixie cups and freeze for 6 hours to overnight.
   Makes about 4-6 pops

The Best Part of Pie

3 nectarines or any fruit
1 T. butter
Small handful of walnuts
Optional: 1 scant T. pure maple syrup

1. Chop fruit.
2. Melt butter in pan over medium heat.
3. Add fruit and walnuts and stir.
4. Cook until fruit is soft, which brings out its natural sweetness. If you are using maple syrup, stir into the mixture and serve. *Serves 1*

Orange and Coconut Treat

4 oranges, peeled and cut into segments
2 bananas, peeled and sliced
½ cup shredded unsweetened coconut
2 T. sliced, toasted almonds

1. Prepare fruit and toss with coconut and almonds.

   Serves 1

Toxicity and Inflammation Quiz

TOXICITY AND INFLAMMATION QUIZ

Quiz based on Dr. Mark Hyman's book "The UltraSimple Diet"

As you complete the quiz, be completely honest with yourself. It is a good indicator of how toxic you really are. You should take the quiz during the Prep Week before you begin the 21-days of the Refresh and again during the Post Week phase. If you suffer from any of the symptoms in the quiz, my hope is that this Refresh will assist you in getting on the right track in regaining your health.

You will be surprised how many of your symptoms disappear In this short period of time.

The forms on the following pages will make it easy to keep track of your scores.

Fill out the Before column now, and then the After column at the end of the Refresh. Then record the Differences in your scores in the column on the far right. The first time you take the quiz, please rate each of the following symptoms based upon your health profile for the last 30 days.

USE THE FOLLOWING SCALE TO RATE YOUR SYMPTONS:

0 = *Never or almost never have the symptom*

1 = *Occasionally have it, effect is not severe*

2 = *Occasionally have it, effect is severe*

3 = *Frequently have it, effect is not severe*

4 = *Frequently have it, effect is severe*

DIGESTIVE TRACT:	Before	After	Difference
Nausea or vomiting			
Diarrhea			
Constipation			
Belching or passing gas			
Heartburn			
Intestinal / stomach pain			
Subtotal			

EARS:	Before	After	Difference
Itchy ears			
Earaches or ear infections			
Drainage from ear			
Ringing in ears or hearing loss			
Subtotal			

EMOTIONS:	Before	After	Difference
Mood swings			
Anxiety, fear, or nervousness			

Anger, irritability, or aggressiveness			
Depression			
Subtotal			

ENERGY/ACTIVITY:	**Before**	**After**	**Difference**
Fatigue or sluggishness			
Apathy or lethargy			
Hyperactivity			
Restlessness			
Subtotal			

EYES:	**Before**	**After**	**Difference**
Watery or itchy eyes			
Swollen, reddened, or sticky eyelids			
Bags or dark circles under eyes			
Blurred or tunnel vision (does not include near-or far-sightedness)			
Subtotal			

HEAD:	**Before**	**After**	**Difference**
Headaches			
Faintness			
Dizziness			
Insomnia			
Subtotal			

HEART:	**Before**	**After**	**Difference**
Irregular or skipped heartbeat			
Rapid or pounding heartbeat			
Chest pain			
Subtotal			

JOINTS/MUSCLES:	**Before**	**After**	**Difference**
Aches or pain in joints			
Arthritis			
Stiffness or limitation of movement			
Aches or pain in muscles			

Feeling of weakness or tiredness			
Subtotal			

LUNGS:	Before	After	Difference
Chest congestion			
Asthma or bronchitis			
Shortness of breath			
Difficulty breathing			
Subtotal			

MIND:	Before	After	Difference
Poor memory			
Confusion or poor comprehension			
Poor concentration			
Poor physical coordination			
Difficulty making decisions			
Stuttering or stammering			
Slurred speech			

Learning disabilities			
Subtotal			

MOUTH/THROAT:	Before	After	Difference
Chronic coughing			
Gagging or frequent need to clear throat			
Sore throat, hoarseness, or loss of voice			
Swollen or discolored tongue, gum, or lips			
Canker sores			
Subtotal			

NOSE:	Before	After	Difference
Stuffy nose			
Sinus problems			
Hay fever			
Sneezing attacks			
Excessive mucus formation			
Subtotal			

SKIN:	**Before**	**After**	**Difference**
Acne			
Hives, rashes, or dry skin			
Hair loss			
Flushing or hot flushes			
Excessive sweating			
Subtotal			

WEIGHT:	**Before**	**After**	**Difference**
Binge eating / drinking			
Craving certain foods			
Excessive weight			
Compulsive eating			
Water retention			
Skip meals often			
Excess alcohol intake			
Night eating			
Subtotal			

OTHER:	**Before**	**After**	**Difference**
Frequent illness			
Frequent or urgent urination			
Genital itching or discharge			
Subtotal			

GRAND TOTAL			

ASSESSMENT KEY TO QUIZ

Add your individual scores and subtotal each section. Add the section scores and put your grand total in the Before column. Then check the following to assess the level of your health problems and the potential health benefits of the Attain True Health Refresh.

10 or less (Optimal Health) *Potential Benefits:* Increased energy, improved mood, and weight loss.

11-50 (Mild Imbalance) In addition to the above *Potential Benefits* , you may also see improved digestion, better skin, and less nasal congestion.

51-100 (Moderate Imbalance) You may experience all of the above *Potential Benefits* as well as reduced joint pain, muscle aches, headaches, and more.

Over 100 (Severe Imbalance) You may experience much of the above *Potential Benefits* but to deeply address your chronic symptoms, you might need my support in following a 6-month program that will allow you to better address your overall eating habits and lifestyle imbalances.

TAKE YOUR VITALS

Although the focus of the Attain True Health Spring Cleanse is to detoxify your body, it is important to know where you have begun and where you finish in other areas as well. So I suggest you take your measurements before the Cleanse begins.

MEASUREMENTS:	**Before**	**After**	**Difference**
Weight (in pounds)			
Waist* (in inches)			
Hips** (in inches)			
BMI*** (see below)			

*Take your waist measurement by wrapping a tape measure around your back, side and over your belly button.

** Measure your hips at the widest point, which should be right below the bones of your pelvis and around your bottom.

*** Body Mass Index (BMI) is a number calculated from a person's weight and height. BMI is a fairly reliable indicator of body fatness for most people. BMI does not measure body fat directly, but research has shown that BMI correlates to direct measures of body fat. Some doctors use this as a diagnostic tool to access your health risk. For our purposes, it is just a good number to know so that we can see if you have lost any body fat (besides pounds) over the 21 day Refresh. The use of BMI allows us to compare your own weight status to that of the general population by using the chart below.

BMI Weight Status per US Government Regulations

Below 18.5	Underweight
18.5 – 24.9	Normal
25.0 – 29.9	Overweight
30.0 and Above	Obese

To calculate your BMI, go to: www.bmicalculator.cc/

Product Ordering

REFRESH ENHANCEMENTS

I am highly recommending a group of products that will enhance your Attain True Health Body and Mind Refresh experience. These products are provided by my brand partner, the Shaklee Corporation—the #1 global, natural nutrition company. I have been doing this Refresh for years and the benefits of these products to enhance the Refresh have been proven:

80% of participants experienced improved energy levels and decreased cravings
72% of participants felt improvements in hunger management
60% of participants felt improvements in mood
74% of participants felt improvement in quality of sleep and mental clarity
96% of participants lost weight

These products will aid in the detoxification process in five ways:

- Improved digestive health
- Enhanced liver support
- Addition of more healthy bacteria to build your gut flora
- Improved immune system
- Jumpstart for weight management

There are several reasons why I recommend the Shaklee products above so many of the other brands available. Let me give you some background information about the Shaklee Corporation. It was founded by Dr. Forrest Shaklee in 1956 after Dr. Shaklee spent years investigating nutrients found in foods and formulating the very first multi-vitamin in 1915. He felt strongly that most of the problems in American health were directly related to poor nutrition and that nutritional intervention would be the most effective way to get people feeling better and on the road to better health. It's amazing that over 100 years later, this is still the case and I feel the same way!

One of Dr. Shaklee's biggest commitments was to forwarding scientific progress. Right from the start, he used scientific experimentation to determine the best combinations of nutrients. Today, the Shaklee Corporation sponsors more scientific research published in peer-reviewed journals than the rest of the natural-nutrition industry combined (and there are over 4000 companies in the US alone marketing nutritional supplements). The products themselves are based on scientific research, as well. They spend over $300 million a year in research and development.

Another reason for my comfort with Shaklee's products is the consistent quality control testing they complete. They test raw materials before production for different contaminants including molds, heavy metals, insecticides and pesticides. And they test during production (the multivitamins are subjected to over 350 quality tests per batch, every time). And then finished products are also tested for potency before shipping. This company does more quality tests on its products than the rest of the natural nutrition industry, over 100,000 tests annually. None of this is required by the government or any regulating body. The Shaklee Corporation does this because it's good business and good for our customers. One fact in my research is that shipments of botanical ingredients rejected by Shaklee are routinely bought by other supplement companies to be used to manufacture their products.

The products are made without any artificial sweeteners, flavors, colors, additives or preservatives. High-performance Olympic athletes use Shaklee products because they know they won't be testing positive for performance-enhancing substances in the tests they need to take when they compete. And NASA has contracted Shaklee to make products for our US astronauts.

From a purely practical standpoint, it's important to know that Shaklee has a 100% money-back guarantee. If for any reason you do not like the product purchased, you can return it for a full refund.

And one more consideration in my decision to use the Shaklee products was their focus on protecting the environment. Shaklee has a commitment to minimizing the impact of the company's business on our planet. Activities such as recycling, using reusable packaging (for instance only the carbon-block insert in the water filter needs to be changed, everything else is reusable), using solar power and planting trees help make Shaklee friendly to the environment. They are also the first ever Climate Neutral certified company in the world, offsetting all their carbon omissions.

I am proud to represent a company where integrity, quality and social responsibility are the standards, and where making people and the planet healthier is their mission. Shaklee is all about helping people take control of your future health by virtue of your choices today. Shaklee products – and the quality and science behind them – are unmatched in the industry.

With that being said, here is a list of my recommendations to enhance your Refresh experience:

It is advisable to order your products during the Preparation Week so that they will be available for the start of the 21 days. These recommendations will only enhance your Refresh experience and beyond. All products can be ordered here: **www.attaintruehealthsolutions.com**
Member Prices entitle you to a 15% discount. Please see page 263 for more details of the Member Pricing designated by asterisks in the price lists.

PRODUCTS FOR THE REFRESH:

1. **Shaklee Life Energizing Shake**

   This delicious protein powder contains nutrients clinically proven to help create the foundation for a longer, healthier life. They are designed to increase your energy, help you achieve a healthier weight and provide incredible digestive and immune support from fiber and probiotics. Available in soy and non-soy formulas.

   The Shaklee Life Energizing Shake protein powder comes packed with:

- 24 grams of plant-based, non-GMO protein
- Added leucine to help preserve lean muscle and achieve a healthier weight
- A powerful combination of prebiotics and 1 billion CFU of probiotics
- Omega-3 (ALA) to support heart and brain health

The Life Shake is also gluten free, lactose free, low glycemic, and Kosher. And contains no added artificial flavors, sweeteners or preservatives

You may order 2 canisters, which make 15 smoothies each and this way you get to pick two flavors for a variety of smoothie options. Or you can order one flavor in a 30-day pouch. Flavors choices are chocolate, strawberry, vanilla and café latte. Recipes are provided in the Recipe section.

Depending upon which size and version (soy or non-soy) you order, the prices will vary. (all item #'s can found on my Shaklee website. Ordering instructions on page 252.)

Member Prices vary from: $40-$100*
Retail Prices vary from $62 - $117

2. Healthy Cleanse Supplement Regimen (comes as a bundle) The bundle contains:

a) Alfalfa Complex
Alfalfa is nature's powerhouse! It is a cooling, sweet, astringent herb that cleanses toxins from tissues and naturally lowers your cholesterol. Its roots can grow 20 feet down into the earth making it very rich in minerals and Vitamins A, D, E, and K, as well as chlorophyll. Chlorophyll is a natural compound that modern research has shown to be useful as an agent in the fight against cancer, stroke, heart disease and diabetes. Alfalfa Complex is a perfect aid to the introduction of all 'real' foods and will be integral for the initiation into the process of our body's own natural detoxification.

b) Liver DTX
Our liver is our main detoxification organ. We are trying to clean and rejuvenate our liver during the Refresh, to allow it to work more efficiently. This supplement actually contains milk thistle (shown to support the body's normal ability to regenerate liver cells), reishi mushrooms (which are high in antioxidant qualities), dandelion greens, turmeric and artichoke (all natural detoxifiers). This supplement will enhance the 'cleaning' of your liver.

c) Herb Lax
Encourages a mild cleansing action to aid the body's natural processes.

d) Optiflora Probiotic Complex
Helps promote healthy intestinal activity and good digestive health. Adds in 1 million extra probiotics that utilize patented triple-layer encapsulation technology which is designed for live delivery of the probiotics to the large intestine, where they provide the greatest benefit.

#89413
Member Price: $79.70
Retail price: $93.70

OPTIONAL PRODUCTS FOR THE REFRESH BUT HIGHLY RECOMMENDED:

1. Multi Vitamin (Pick one of 3 choices)

a. Shaklee Life Strip (Best Option!)
Every serving of Shaklee Life Strip is the culmination of years of research and quality testing to guarantee Shaklee delivers pure and potent vitamins, minerals, omega-3 fatty acids, polyphenols, antioxidants and phytonutrients to help create the foundation for a longer, healthier life. This comprehensive nutrition system contains:

- Vivix® Liquigels for Cellular Health; Healthy Aging
  Triple patented, all natural blend of a broad spectrum of polyphenols with key ingredients shown in laboratory studies to protect and repair DNA and combat free radicals.
- OmegaGuard® Plus for Heart Health; Brain Health
  One gram of pure, ultra-concentrated DHA/EPA omega-3 fatty acids, combined with heart-healthy CoQ10 and Vitamin E in an enteric-coated softgel to eliminate fishy aftertaste.
- Advanced Multivitamin for Complete Nutrition; Bone and Joint Health
  Provides over 100% DV of essential vitamins. Dissolves in less than 30 minutes in the stomach and is designed to enhance absorption of folic acid from the patented microcoating.
- B+C Complex for Immune Health; Energy
  Provides over 100% DV of essential vitamins. Dissolves in less than 30 minutes in the stomach and is designed to enhance absorption of folic acid from the patented micro-coating.

With Iron –#21294
Without Iron –#21293
Member Price: $169.96*
Retail Price: $200.00

b. Shaklee Vitalizer (Great Option)
Vitalizer is supplementation made simple. Our unique, clinically supported solution packs essential nutrition into a

convenient, everyday, go-anywhere Vita-Strip®. Designed to enhance absorption, Vitalizer provides vitamins, minerals, antioxidants, omega-3s, and healthy probiotics—all in one Vitalizer Vita-Strip®.
It has a patented delivery system designed to enhance absorption of key nutrients.

Vitalizer supports optimal health and promotes:

- Heart health
- Bone and Joint health
- Immune health
- Digestive health
- Brain and vision health
- Physical energy

Women's –#20283
Men's –#20282
Gold (for over age 50) –#20284
Member Prices vary from $79.29-84.95*
Retail Prices vary from $93.25-$100

c. Shaklee Vita Lea (Good Option)
Vita-Lea is a high-potency formulation specially designed to support our unique needs. Each serving delivers 100% or more of the Daily Value of all vitamins, including twice the Daily Value of vitamins C, D, and E—plus beta-carotene for safely increasing antioxidant protection. It comes in iron or non-iron formulas

Vita Lea supports optimal health and promotes:
- Heart health
- Immune health
- Bone and joint health
- Physical energy
- Healthy skin, hair, and nails

With Iron –#20288
Without Iron –#20286
Member Price: $23.05*
Retail Price: $27.10

2. Shaklee 'Get Clean' Line of Cleaning Products

Environmentally-friendly, non-toxic, green cleaning supplies for your home (found under Healthy Home on the website). We will be reducing the toxic load so it is recommended to eliminate the cleaning supplies that have toxins in them that you will be breathing.

3. Shaklee Enfuselle Skin Care Line

An all-natural skin care line that fights against cellular aging and reduces the toxin load with no parabens, phthalates etc. (found under Healthy Beauty on the website)–less toxins seeping into the pours of your skin.

4. Shaklee 'Get Clean' Water Pitcher

Our naturally alkalizing water pitcher, also found in the Get Clean line (another way to alkalize your pH) is made with the highest-quality natural ingredients available!

All of these products can be found by the putting product name or # in the search bar on the website:
www.attaintruehealthsolutions.com

OPTIONAL SUPPLEMENT BUNDLES FOR SPECIFIC HEALTH CONCERNS:

Consider my recommendations for high quality natural supplements for relief and recovery. Sourced by nature, proven by science and personally researched and tested on a variety of my clients!

Allergies:
NutriFeron (#20962)
Alfalfa Complex (#20153)
Vitamin C (#20095)

Stress/Anxiety:
Stress Relief Complex (#20656)
B-Complex (#20186)
Vivix (#21500)

Arthritis/Joint Pain:
Joint Health (#20281)
OsteoMatrix (#21217)
Alfalfa Complex(#20153)

Digestion/IBS/Crohns:
OptiFlora (#20639)
EZ-Gest (Digestive Enzymes) (#20633)
NutriFeron (#20962)

Energy:
B-Complex (#20186)
Stress Relief Complex (#20656)
Core Energy (#20732)

Fibromyalgia:
Vitamin D3(#21214)
OsteoMatrix (#21217)
Liver DTX (#20616)
Alfalfa Complex (#20153)
Lecithin (#20182)
Life Strip (#21293)

Hypoglycemia/Pre-Diabetes:
Glucose Regulation(#20749)
Alfalfa Complex (#20153)
Vivix (#21500)

Inflammation:
Vivix (#21500)
Alfalfa Complex (#20153)
NutriFeron (#20962)
Life Strip (#21293)

Immunity:
Immunity Formula 1(#20241)
NutriFeron (#20962),
Vitalized Immunity (#22073)
Vitamin D3 (#21214)

Mental Clarity/Focus/Memory:
Mind Works (#22066)
Vivix (#21500))
Vitalizer (#20284)

Menopause:
Menopause Balance (#20645)
GLA Complex (#20608)
Vitamin D3 (#21214)

PMS Symptoms:
GLA Complex (#20608)
Stress Relief Complex (#20656))
B-Complex (#20186))

Sleep:
Gentle Sleep Complex (#20603)
Cal Mag Complex (#21216)
Stress Relief(#20656)

Thyroid/Hashimotos:
Stress Relief Complex (#20656)
Glucose Regulation Complex (#20749)
Life Strip (#21213)

HOW TO ORDER YOUR SHAKLEE SUPPLEMENTS

As part of the **Attain True Health Body and Mind Refresh**, it is recommended that you order the Shaklee Life Shake and Healthy Cleanse Bundle (at a minimum) by placing your order online at: **www.attaintruehealthsolutions.com**

Any of the other optional products such as a multi-vitamin, the Get Clean healthy home products and our all-natural skin care line are also great options during the Refresh.

NOTE: *The use of products is encouraged but please check with your healthcare provider if you have any questions about the use of supplementation and protein powders and what may be best for your overall health.*

You will continue to take them all for 30 days and I encourage you to continue with these long after the Refresh is over.

**During the ordering process, the website asks if you would like to become a 'member' or just order as a guest. Be aware that you may order these products without becoming a member or paying any additional fees. However, if you do choose to become a 'member' for either $19.95 (one-time fee for life) or free membership depending upon the product regimen you order - the advantages are endless (and healthy) and most importantly, there is a 15% discount on all products. I am encouraging you to join as a member since there is substantial savings and you will most certainly want to continue with the protein powder long after the Refresh is over since it is a most convenient breakfast option.*
PLEASE NOTE: I understand that some of us are apprehensive about ordering supplements when we do not know how they will affect us. Please be assured that I have tested the Shaklee products and find them to be of the highest quality and manufactured with integrity and all natural ingredients. **And...there is a 100% money- back guarantee!**

Made in the USA
Middletown, DE
13 January 2017